SENSATIONAL PRESERVES

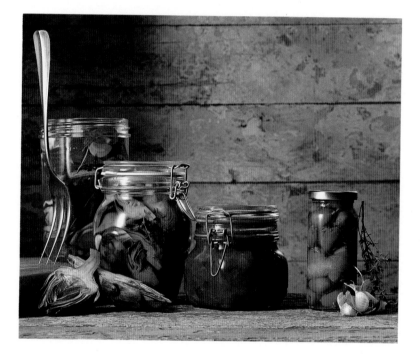

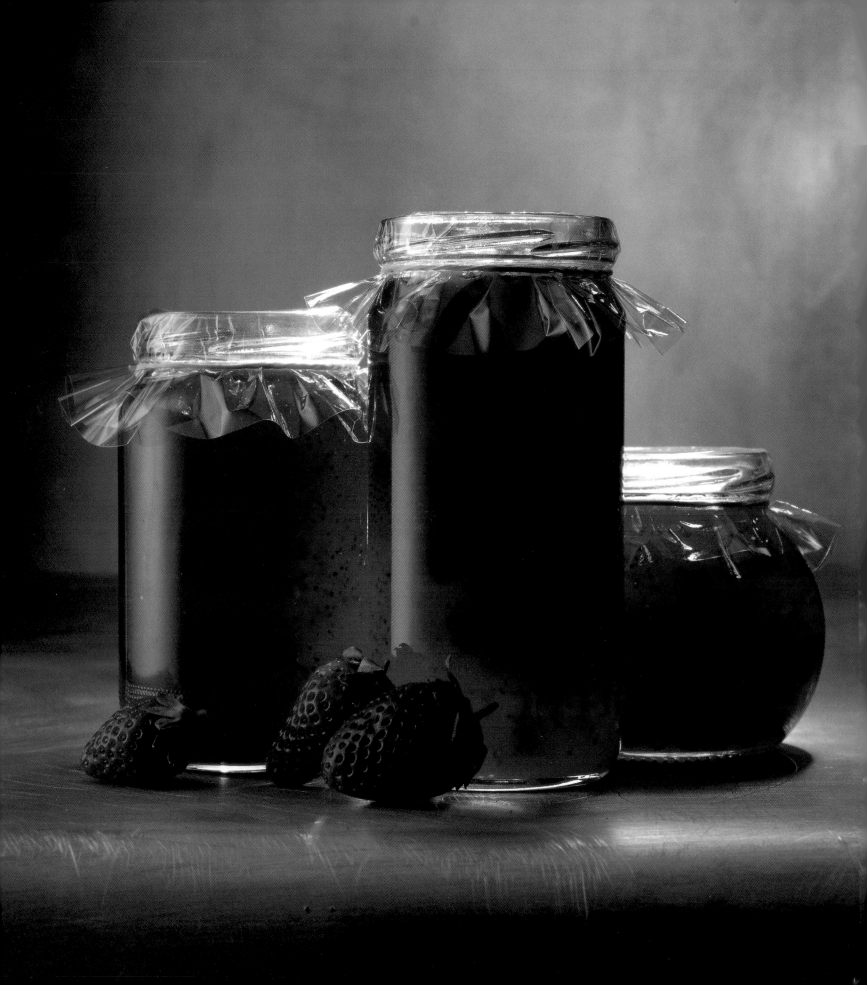

SENSATIONAL PRESERVES

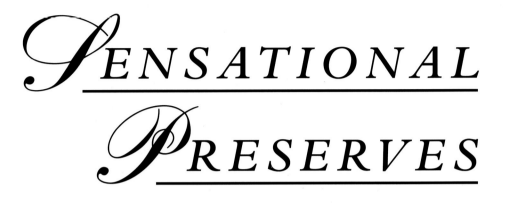

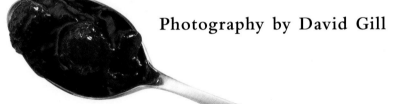

HILAIRE WALDEN

Photography by David Gill

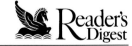
Reader's Digest

The Reader's Digest Association, Inc.
Pleasantville, New York/Montreal

A Reader's Digest Book

Designed and edited by Conran Octopus Limited

The credits and acknowledgments that appear on page 144
are hereby made a part of this copyright page.

First published in Great Britain in 1995 by Conran Octopus Limited

Library of Congress Cataloging in Publication Data
Walden, Hilaire.
    Sensational preserves / Hilaire Walden ; photography by David
      Gill.
        p.   cm.
    Includes index.
    ISBN 0-89577-840-8
    1. Fruit—Preservation. 2. Vegetables—Preservation. I. Title.
TX612.F7W25   1996
641.4—dc20   95-25974

COMMISSIONING EDITOR: Sarah Pearce
PROJECT EDITOR: Charlotte Coleman-Smith
ART EDITOR: Sue Storey
COPY EDITOR: Beverly Le Blanc
HOME ECONOMIST: Meg Jansz
PHOTOGRAPHIC STYLIST: Hilary Guy
PRODUCTION: Clare Coles
INDEX: Hilary Bird

Printed in Hong Kong

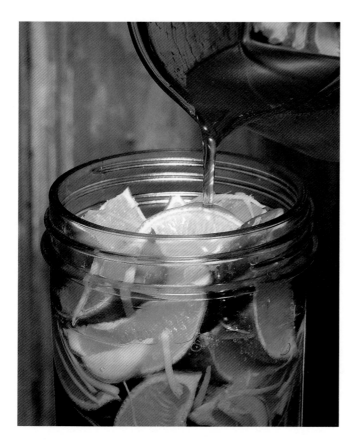

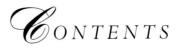

CONTENTS

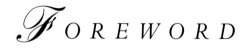OREWORD

Preserves add enormous variety to cooking and eating and provide an endless wealth of ideas, whether you want to make a quick snack, add a new twist to a main course, or perhaps create an unusual dessert. They can be used as accompaniments for both sweet and savory dishes, in sauces, salad dressings and drinks, and even in casseroles and sorbets.

Preserves solve many a gift-giving problem. A beribboned bottle or jar of homemade preserves is always well received and is one of the most cost-effective ways of making your own gifts.

Although there is a wide and cosmopolitan variety of commercial products available, it does not match the varied selection you can make in your own home. The feeling of satisfaction from having prepared a batch of crimson strawberry conserve or glowing amber jam to put by for the autumn can't be denied. Neither can the gratification of seeing a row of homemade preserves lined up in your pantry.

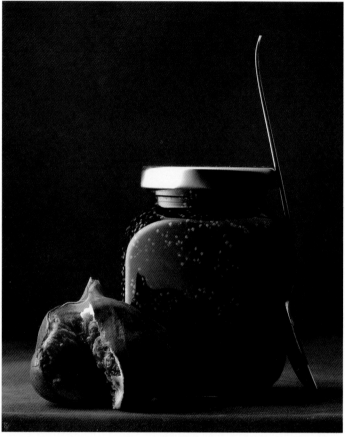

Above: This superb Fig Conserve (see page 93) is one of the many exotic preserves that are easily made at home.

You will find that making preserves is easy; many recipes can be made by novice and experienced cooks alike. The equipment is very basic, and you probably already have all that is needed in your own kitchen. If you do not have access to homegrown fruit and vegetables, find a good farmer's market or spend a few hours pick your own at specially designated orchards and fields. There is no need to make preserves in vast quantities, so I have deliberately kept quantities practical and relevant.

In this book you will find recipes for preserves from around the world. You can also have fun blending spices and combining fruits and vegetables to make your own unique creations, whether you want an unusual flavor or something less exotic.

ESSENTIAL INGREDIENTS

PECTIN is a natural gumlike substance found in the cells of fruit. Pectin is extracted from fruit by acid (also present in the fruit) during cooking, and when cooked with sugar, it produces a set. Underripe fruit contains more pectin than ripe fruit.

Pectin Content of Fruits

High	Medium	Low
Black currants	Eating apples	Bananas
Cooking apples	Apricots	Blueberries
Crab apples	Blackberries	Cherries
Cranberries	Figs	Elderberries
Gooseberries	Grapes	Guavas
Lemons	Loganberries	Mangoes
Limes	Mulberries	Melons
Oranges,	Plums	Nectarines
esp. Seville	Raspberries	Peaches
Plums		Pineapples
(some varieties)		Rhubarb
Quinces		Strawberries
Red currants		

Fruits that are very low in pectin are usually combined with a high-pectin fruit or with lemon juice. Liquid pectin can also be used, or you can make your own pectin extract (see below).

Ready-to-use commercial fruit pectins: Made from apples or citrus fruits, these can be quickly substituted for homemade pectin in jam and jelly recipes. Look for liquid commercial pectin in your local supermarket. Use one 3-ounce pouch (or half of a 6-ounce bottle) for every ⅔ cup homemade pectin called for in the recipe. Then follow the manufacturer's directions for preparing the jam or jelly.

Testing for pectin and making pectin extract: Chop 2 pounds apple peelings and cores (or whole sour cooking apples or crab apples), cover with 4½ cups water, and simmer gently, stirring occasionally, for about 45 minutes or until pulpy. Pour the contents of the pan into a scalded jelly bag suspended over a large bowl (see page 17) and leave to drain, undisturbed, in a cool place for 8–12 hours. Put 1 teaspoon of the strained juice in a jar and add 1 tablespoon grain alcohol. Cover the jar and shake it, then leave to stand for 5 minutes. If a jellylike clot forms (pectin extract), then the juice has a good pectin content. This test can also be used to test the pectin content of fruit after it has had its first cooking. Store the pectin extract in the refrigerator once you have made it. Use 1¼ cups of the extract for every 4 pounds low-pectin fruit and add it to the fruit after it has been cooked but before the sugar is added.

ACID is either naturally present in fruit or can be added in the form of citric acid or lemon juice. It is essential for a good set. The acid level in fruits declines as they ripen, which is why slightly underripe fruits are often recommended. Wild or late-season cultivated blackberries, as well as strawberries, pears, eating apples, cherries, and vegetables such as summer squash, all need additional acid. Allow ½ teaspoon citric acid or 2 tablespoons lemon juice for every 4 pounds low-pectin fruit.

SUGAR is needed for preservation, for flavor and for setting jams, jellies, marmalades, and conserves (these preserves must contain sufficient sugar, pectin, and acid in order to set). The more pectin a fruit contains, the more sugar it will set. If fruit has a high pectin content, 3⅓ cups sugar can be added to 1 pound fruit (1½ times the weight of the fruit). Fruit with a medium pectin content will need an equal weight of sugar. If fruit has a low pectin content, acid and pectin must be added, as well as an equal quantity of sugar to fruit.

It is important to use the right amount of sugar to make sure a preserve will set. Too little sugar will result in fermentation; too much will hinder setting and may cause crystallization.

If sugar is added to a preserve before the fruit is really soft, the fruit will harden and no amount of cooking will tenderize it. This hardening effect can be used deliberately. If, for example, you want very soft fruit such as strawberries and raspberries to remain whole, sprinkle them with sugar and leave overnight before cooking.

Granulated sugar is most widely used for sweet preserves.

Brown sugar can be used for sweet preserves, but it takes longer to dissolve and affects the color and flavor of the preserve. Brown sugar is more often used for savory preserves.

Honey has a distinctive flavor and should be substituted only for a small proportion of the sugar. Honey can hinder the ability of a preserve to reach setting point.

Warming sugar: Sugar will dissolve more quickly if it is warm. Put the required amount of sugar in a heatproof bowl, then place in an oven preheated to the lowest setting for about 20 minutes or until the sugar is warm but not hot.

SALT Table salt is not suitable (except for brining pickles), as it contains additives to keep it free-flowing; these can cause discoloration and may inhibit some preservative qualities. Instead, use pure rock salt or kosher salt.

VINEGAR I prefer to use red or white wine vinegars because they have a more subtle flavor than ordinary white distilled vinegar. Cider vinegar is used in making fruity chutneys and relishes.

Types of Preserves

JAM A thick, sweet preserve containing pieces of fruit or whole fruits, such as strawberries. It should hold its shape well without being too runny or too solid.
WATCHPOINTS See *Making Jams* (pages 14–15)
Sugar-reduced jam: The quantity of sugar should not be reduced by more than 20 percent or the jam will be runny and will not keep for more than 3–4 weeks in a cool place or 6 weeks in a refrigerator.
Freezer jam: This is quick to make and has a fresh taste and a softer set than conventional jams. The fruit is not cooked in this type of preserve. To help achieve a set, liquid pectin or pectin extract (see page 7) is added. Freezer jam must be kept in the refrigerator after thawing.

JELLY A preserve made from fruit juice that is tender, yet firm enough to hold its shape. By convention, jellies should be crystal clear, but the clarity depends on slow, undisturbed straining of the cooked unsweetened fruit. The amount of water used affects the strength of flavor of the prepared jelly.
WATCHPOINTS See *Making Jellies* (pages 16–17)

Below, from left to right: Plum Jelly, Seville Orange Marmalade, Strawberry Conserve, Pecan and Whiskey Mincemeat, Lemon Curd.

MARMALADE A sweet preserve based on citrus fruits. Seville oranges make the best marmalades; sweet oranges tend to give a more cloudy appearance and their pith does not become translucent. Marmalades can be chunky, thin-cut, or fine-shred.
WATCHPOINTS See *Making Marmalades* (pages 18–19)

CONSERVE Made from whole or chopped fruit suspended in a thick or lightly set syrup. The fruit, which must be completely dry, is layered with sugar and left overnight to coax the juices out and keep the fruit firm. The subsequent brief boiling draws out more juices, often making it unnecessary to add any water. The short cooking time preserves the fresh, fruity flavor.
WATCHPOINTS See *Making Jams* (pages 14–15)

FRUIT BUTTER A soft, thick, spreadable mixture of sieved fruit purée and sugar. The texture is determined by consistency rather than by set or temperature. The fruit is cooked with a minimum of water until soft, then puréed and sieved through a nonmetallic sieve; 1¼–1¾ cups sugar is added to every 1 pound fruit pulp, and the mixture is heated gently, then boiled for 30–45 minutes or until the butter has the consistency of sour cream. Stir the mixture occasionally at first, then more frequently as the cooking progresses. To test for correct consistency, put a spoonful on a cold plate; if water seeps out, the butter is too thin and should be cooked longer.
WATCHPOINTS For making fruit butter
- *Caramelized butter:* The purée was too thin before the sugar was added and before sufficient water had evaporated. Discard.
- *Thin, flavorless butter:* The butter was insufficiently cooked and may ferment on storage. Boil a little longer to thicken.

FRUIT SPREAD A fruit butter that has been cooked for 45–55 minutes or until it is so thick that it sets firmly enough to be sliced. Fruit spreads can be set in decorative molds.
WATCHPOINTS See *Fruit Butter*

FRUIT CURD Made from egg yolks or whole eggs, sugar, and fruit or fruit juice. Use fresh, free-range eggs and unsalted butter.
WATCHPOINTS For making fruit curd
- *Curdling eggs:* The bottom of the basin touched the water during cooking; the water was boiling rather than simmering. To remedy, transfer the basin immediately to a bowl of cold water and beat the curd vigorously. Strain through a nonmetallic sieve and start again, adding another egg.

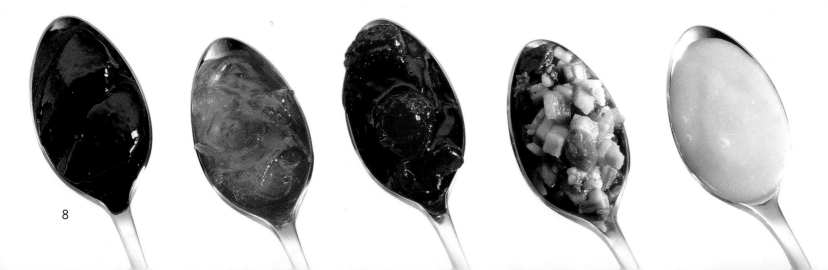

TYPES OF PRESERVES

MINCEMEAT This was originally made with ground meat. In today's mixtures the meat has been replaced by beef suet. Vegetarian suets are also available.

WATCHPOINTS For making mincemeat
- *Fermentation:* There is insufficient sugar, fruit, acid, or alcohol in the mincemeat; the jars are not clean. Rectify by reboiling the mincemeat (although it may soften and the flavor may be affected).
- *Dry surface:* The mincemeat was not covered properly. Stir in a little of the alcohol used in the recipe and cover again.

FRUITS IN ALCOHOL Raw or lightly cooked fruit is steeped in alcohol. Any spirit or liqueur that is at least 40 percent alcohol (80 proof) will be effective. Wines and fortified wines need to be combined with another means of preservation, usually sugar.

WATCHPOINTS For making fruits in alcohol
- *Fruit rises to top of jar:* Weight down with crumpled waxed paper. Remove after 1 week and top up with alcohol.

CANDIED, CRYSTALLIZED, AND GLACE FRUITS A selection of fruits is impregnated with sugar over a period of about 3 weeks and then air-dried.

WATCHPOINTS See *Making Candied Fruits* (pages 20–21)

Below, from left to right: Quince Spread, Tomato Ketchup, Dill Pickled Gherkins, Mango Chutney, and Beet and Horseradish Relish.

CHUTNEY A sweet-sour mixture of coarsely chopped vegetables and fruit cooked with spices or herbs, vinegar, and sugar. You can use bruised vegetables if you remove the affected parts, but avoid moldy produce. Fruit should not be overripe. Thick-skinned fruit or vegetables should be cooked first in the vinegar to soften them. The fruit or vegetables are cooked slowly with the remaining ingredients until the mixture is smooth and thick, with no free liquid. The chutney should be stirred frequently.

WATCHPOINTS For making chutney
- *Dry, brown surface:* The cover is not airtight; the storage place is too warm. Discard.
- *Fermenting or moldy chutney:* The storage place is too warm; there is insufficient vinegar or sugar; the chutney is too thin; the jars or lids are dirty. Discard.

RELISH Similar to a chutney but containing smaller pieces of vegetables or fruit. Relishes have a shorter cooking time.

WATCHPOINTS See *Chutney* (above).

SAUCE Bottled sauces were popular in 19th- and early 20th-century England. The word *ketchup* comes from the Far East and traditionally was applied to thin, salty sauces. After cooking in a spiced vinegar, the vegetables or fruits are sieved or puréed, then simmered to a creamy consistency.

WATCHPOINTS For making sauces
- *Thin sauce:* The sauce was not boiled long enough and may spoil.

PICKLES Raw or lightly cooked vegetables or fruits are preserved in clear spiced vinegar. Raw vegetables are usually salted before being pickled, either with dry salt (for wet vegetables such as cucumbers) or in brine. Salting draws out excess moisture, which would dilute the vinegar and shorten the storage time. Salted vegetables must be rinsed under cold running water, then drained and dried thoroughly. Cooked vegetables do not need brining but should be dried thoroughly before cooking. Fruits are lightly cooked in sweetened spiced vinegar; the vinegar can be boiled to make a syrup.

WATCHPOINTS For making pickles
- *Moldy pickles:* The brining solution was not strong enough; the vinegar was too weak; the jars were not clean; the vegetables are not covered by vinegar. Discard.
- *Cloudy vinegar:* The brining was not done for long enough; ground spices were used.

VEGETABLES IN OIL Surplus water must be removed from vegetables first by cooking them. Choose vegetables that are in good condition and use fresh oil. I use a mild olive oil because it adds a richness of flavor (it is a good idea to open a new bottle).

WATCHPOINTS For making vegetables in oil
- *Rancid oil:* The storage place is too warm or light; the oil was not fresh. Discard.
- *Moldy or discolored vegetables at top of jar:* The vegetables have not been completely covered in oil; surplus water was not removed from them. Discard.

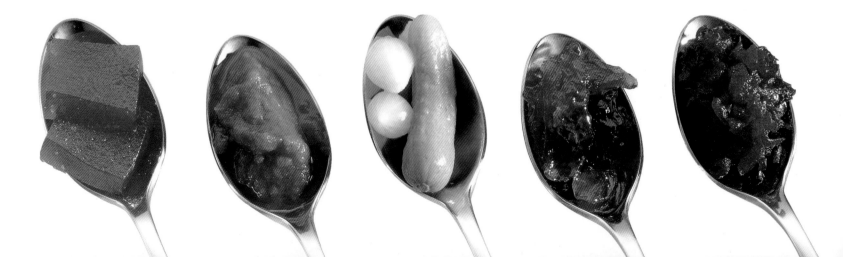

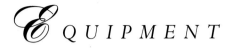QUIPMENT

PAN A traditional preserving pan (maslin) with sloping sides, a pouring lip, and carrying handle is useful but not essential (the recipes in this book are for fairly small amounts).

The pan should not be more than half full when cooking sweetened mixtures, as they spit in hot explosions when boiled. It should provide a large surface area to allow unwanted water to steam and evaporate rapidly; if you are boiling a fairly small quantity of a savory sauce, you can use a large nonstick frying pan.

Make sure your pan is not pitted or damaged in any way. The base should be flat and heavy so that heat is conducted evenly and mixtures do not burn on the bottom of the pan. Stainless steel pans are often recommended, but aluminum pans with nonstick linings are fine. Unlined copper or brass pans should not be used unless specified. Two handles opposite each other make for easy lifting.

KNIVES Stainless steel knives prevent discoloration of fruit and vegetables.

FOOD PROCESSOR Cuts down the time it takes to prepare vegetables and fruit peels.

LONG-HANDLED WOODEN SPOONS Use for all stirring, especially hot mixtures and those containing acid (a metal spoon may react with the acid and discolor the ingredients).

SLOTTED SPOON OR SKIMMER For skimming scum and removing pits from hot mixtures.

SIEVES AND COLANDERS Use heatproof plastic or nylon. These are essential for use with ingredients containing acid.

NONMETALLIC BOWLS Necessary when using ingredients containing acid.

HEATPROOF MEASURING CUPS Essential for measuring and pouring hot mixtures.

WIDE-NECKED NONMETALLIC FUNNEL For pouring liquids from one container into another without spilling.

JELLY BAG A bag shaped like a windsock, usually nylon, used when making jellies. Jelly bags are often sold with their own stand but can easily be fixed to the legs of an upturned stool or suspended from a wire coat hanger hanging from a peg. A nonmetallic bowl placed beneath the bag will catch the drips. A jelly bag can be improvised by tying a double thickness of cheesecloth, muslin, or fine cloth to the legs of an upturned stool. Always scald the jelly bag before use.

CHEESECLOTH BAG To enclose spices or seeds so that they can be removed before the preserve is put into jars. Use cheesecloth, muslin, or fine cloth. Tie the bag to the pan handle with string long enough for it to be suspended in the preserve.

LADLE For transferring preserves from the pan to the containers without spilling.

TONGS For lifting hot bottles and jars.

JARS AND BOTTLES Examine them carefully to make sure there are no cracks, chips, or other flaws. If a hot mixture is added to a flawed jar, the jar will immediately shatter. Bacteria can breed in small cracks, which could cause your preserve to spoil.

For processing in a water bath (see page 13), you will need special jars with lids that are held in place with screw bands or clips. **Preparing jars and bottles:** Wash well in hot soapy water, then rinse and let stand in hot

water until ready to fill. To prevent cracking, use hot jars when filling with hot preserves; cool jars when filling with cold preserves.

COVERS AND LIDS Use acid-proof canning jar covers – each commonly consisting of a metal screw band and a dome metal cap edged with a sealing compound. Other types on the market are dome glass covers with separate rubber sealing rings and metal

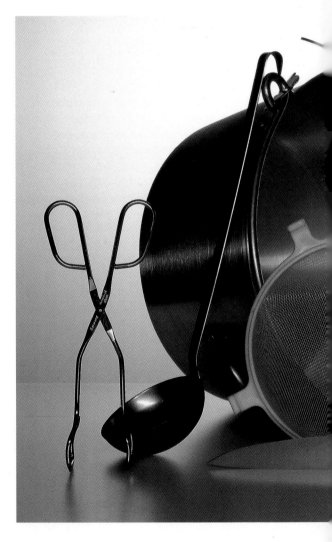

ℰQUIPMENT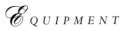

spring clips. Before using, wash in hot soapy water and rinse well. Half-fill a saucepan with water, bring to a simmer, remove from the heat, and slide in the bands, caps, rings and clips. Let stand until ready to use. Metal screw bands may be reused, provided you sterilize them in boiling water for 10 minutes. But discard all metal caps and rubber rings after using them the first time; always use new ones.

When using corks, be sure they are new (do not reuse). Sanitize them in boiling water for 10 minutes to expand them and ensure they are clean.

LABELS Choose labels that have a good adhesive backing and plenty of space for recording important information.

PRESSURE CANNERS When preserving, use a pressure canner – not a pressure cooker – to save processing time and retain the color and flavor of the fruit. A pressure canner is larger than a pressure cooker, holds more canning jars of all different sizes, has a proper rack, and is more reliable in maintaining the proper pressure needed.
1. Remove the trivet from the pan (except for bottling, when it is used upside down).

2. The pan should not be more than half full.
3. When making jams, jellies, and marmalades, cook the fruit at 10 pounds of pressure (medium). Pectin will be destroyed if cooked at 15 pounds of pressure (high).
4. Reduce the pressure to room temperature before opening.

Below, from left to right: Tongs, ladle, preserving pan, nylon sieve, sharp stainless steel knife, stainless steel saucepan, sugar thermometer with clip, slotted spoon, jelly bag, wooden spoons, heatproof glass bowl, funnel with nonstick lining.

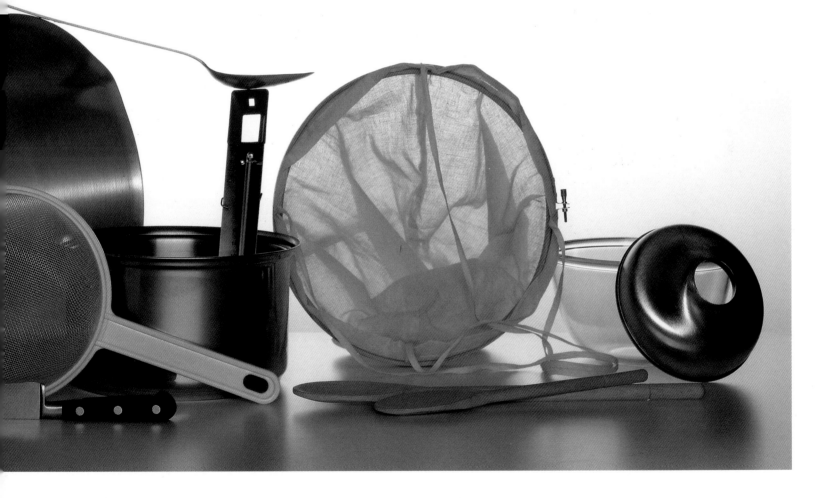

FILLING AND COVERING

To fill containers: For preserves, fill ⅛ inch from the top if sealing with the inversion method and ¼ inch if processing in a water bath; for fruits and tomatoes processed in a water bath, fill ½ inch from the top; for low-acid vegetables and other foods processed in a water bath, fill 1 inch from the top.

All hot preserves should be covered with airtight lids within about 20 minutes. As the preserves cool, so does the air beneath the lid, contracting to create a partial vacuum, which helps to protect the preserves from spoiling. If you have to delay covering the preserves, wait until they are completely cold. If they are covered while lukewarm, the trapped moisture and warmth provide the perfect breeding ground for bacteria and mold.

Jams and conserves: Strawberry jams and conserves should always be left to stand off the heat for 10–15 minutes to prevent fruit rising to the top. For other preserves, see individual recipes (whether preserves are left to stand or not depends on the density of the fruit and the amount used). If in doubt, fill immediately. Ladle into hot, clean, dry jars through a heatproof funnel, then wipe jar rims and threads clean with a hot, soapy cloth. To fill and seal preserves using the inversion method, fill jars up to ⅛ inch from the top. cover with dome metal caps, with sealing compound down next to glass jar rims, and screw the metal bands on tightly. Invert the filled jars for 5 minutes, then turn

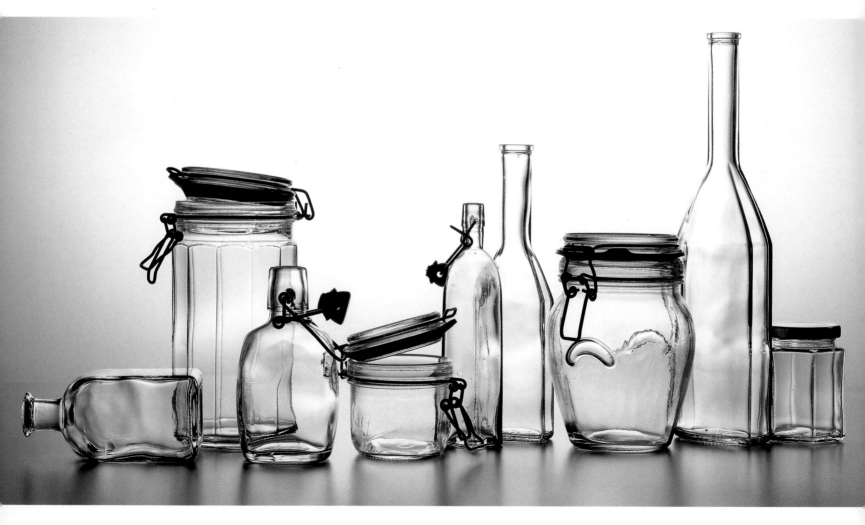

FILLING AND COVERING

upright. Or, if processing by the water bath method, fill jars up to ½ inch from the top. Cover with caps and seal, then process in a simmering water bath (185°F) for 10 minutes (see Processing times, below).

Marmalades: Leave to stand (see individual recipes). Fill, cover, and seal as for jams.

Jellies, fruit butters, curds, and spreads: Can be put into jars immediately (leave jellies to stand if they contain herbs or other particles). Fill, cover, and seal as for jams. To mold a spread, brush the mold lightly first with flavorless oil or cooking spray.

Mincemeat: Leave overnight before putting into jars. Pack in firmly up to ½ inch of the top, leaving no air pockets. Cover and seal as for jams. Process in a pressure canner at 10 pounds pressure for 20 minutes.

Chutneys and relishes: Pour while hot into warm, clean, dry jars up to ½ inch of the tops, leaving no air pockets. Cover with acid-proof lids. Seal as for jams. Process in a simmering-water bath (185°F) for 10 minutes.

Sauces and drinks: Fill containers or bottles while still hot and cover with acid-proof screw-top lids or ground glass stoppers up to ½ inch of the tops. Seal as for jams. Process in a boiling-water bath (212°F) for time specified in the recipe (or 10 minutes if no time is given).

Pickles: Pack the fruit or vegetables into clean, dry jars to within ½ inch of the top, adding any spices as you go; take care when packing cooked vegetables not to ruin their shape. Pour in the vinegar syrup or vinegar (hot for soft pickles such as peaches and prunes, cold for hard ones such as onions), so that the vegetables are well covered, but do not allow the vinegar to come into contact with the lid. Rotate the jar to release trapped air bubbles. Cover with an acid-proof lid. Seal as for jams. Process in a boiling-water bath (212°F) for 10 minutes.

Vegetables in oil and fruits in alcohol: The vegetables or fruits should be completely covered by oil or alcohol up to ½ inch from the top for fruits; 1 inch for vegetables;

rotate the jar to release any trapped air bubbles. Cover fruits in alcohol with acid-proof lids and do not allow the alcohol to touch the lid. Seal vegetables as for jams and process in a boiling-water bath (212°F) for 10 minutes.

Canning fresh fruits: Prepare the fruit and blanche as required. Pack firmly into hot, clean, dry canning jars. Put 1¼ cups sugar in a saucepan with 1¼ cups water and heat gently, stirring, until the sugar has dissolved. Bring to a boil for 1 minute without stirring. Add 1 cup water and return to a boil. If the syrup is not used immediately, cover the pan. The syrup can be flavored with whole spices, freshly grated ginger, or spirits. Pour boiling syrup over the fruit to cover, leaving a headspace of ½ inch to allow for expansion. Process in a water bath at the following temperature and for the times specified. At high altitudes, add 1 minute per 1,000 feet above sea level.

Processing times (pints or quarts): All times refer to processing in a simmering-water bath (185°F) unless specified. Black berries, currants, loganberries, mulberries, raspberries, gooseberries: 2 minutes for normal pack, 10 minutes for tight pack. Whole apricots, cherries, plums: 20 minutes. Halved apricots, nectarines, peaches, plums: 10 minutes. Process whole small peeled peaches in a boiling-water bath (212°F) for 20 minutes.

LABELING Label all containers with contents, date and any storage information.

STORAGE AND SHELF LIFE All preserves should be kept in a cool, dark, dry place.
Jams, jellies, marmalades, and conserves: Will keep for up to 1 year.
Fruit butters: 3 months.
Fruit spreads: Up to 1 year.
Curds: 4–6 weeks in a cool place; 3 months in the refrigerator.
Mincemeat: 12–18 months.
Chutneys and relishes: 1 year or more.

Sauces: See individual recipes.
Drinks: If spirit based, 3–5 years.
Pickles: 1 year or more.
Vegetables in oil: 9–12 months.
Fruits in alcohol: 2 years or more.
Candied, crystallized, and glacé fruits: Up to 2 years, if not longer.

PROCESSING IN A WATER BATH This is a way of extending the shelf-life of canned foods. Air is expelled during processing, creating a partial vacuum in the container. A tight seal is formed, preventing the contents from becoming contaminated. Use flawless canning jars with dome metal caps with a sealing compound and metal screw-bands. A water-bath canner with a tight cover, plus a basket, rack, or trivet is ideal, but a large covered pot works well.

Fill the hot, clean, dry jars, leaving a headspace (see left) to give the food room to expand during processing. As you pack each jar, run a spatula around the inside to remove air bubbles. Cover jars as for jams.

Stand jars securely upright in the basket or on the rack or trivet in the water-bath canner. Check that they are not touching each other or the sides of the pan. Pour in warm water to cover by at least 1 inch; cover the water bath. For jams, jellies, preserves, chutneys, or fruits, bring the water to a simmering temperature (185°F), then begin timing the process. Allow the time specified in the recipe (10 minutes if no time is given). When canning vegetables, sauces, and drinks, heat the water to a boiling temperature (212°F), then process for the time specified in the recipe (10 minutes if no time is given). Be certain the jars stay covered with water during processing and the temperature remains constant.

Transfer the jars with tongs to a wire rack to cool. When cool, check seals by pressing the middle of the lid with your finger. If the lid springs up when your finger is released, the lid is not sealed properly. Refrigerate and use the food within 1 week.

Making Jams

It is best to use fruit that is not quite ripe for making jams, as it contains the most pectin. The amount of sugar that is added will vary according to the sugar content of the fruit (classically, the sugar represents 60–65 percent of the total weight of a finished jam). The longer the fruit takes to cook, the greater the amount of water that is added. The fruit can be gently crushed against the bottom of the pan to quicken the release of the juices (do not crush strawberries, as the pieces should be left whole). The recipe below can be adapted by adding flavorings such as orange-flower water or rosewater, gin, brandy, eau-de-vie, or kirsch. Stir in 2 tablespoons of the flavoring just before putting into jars.

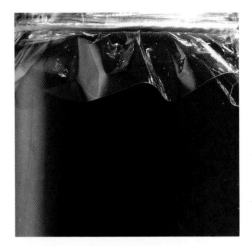

Strawberry Jam

MAKES 5⅓ CUPS

2 pounds strawberries
juice of ½ lemon
⅔ cup pectin extract (see page 7), or 6 ounces
  commercial liquid pectin
4½ cups sugar, warmed (see page 7)
1 tablespoon butter (optional)

EQUIPMENT
• **Sharp stainless steel kitchen knives**
• **Chopping board**
• **Preserving pan or very large nonaluminum**
  saucepan
• **Long-handled wooden spoon**
• **Sugar thermometer (optional)**
• **Saucer and teaspoon**
• **Slotted spoon**
• **Funnel**
• **Suitable jars, lids or covers (see pages 10–11)**

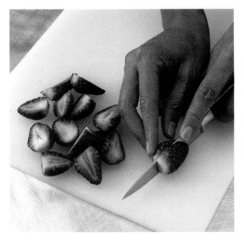

1 Hull and halve the strawberries with a sharp knife. Place them in a large saucepan with the lemon juice and add the pectin extract. (If using commercial pectin, follow the manufacturer's directions.)

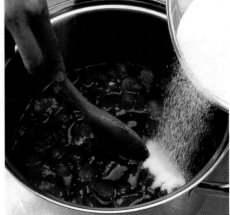

2 Gently warm the contents of the pan over low heat for 3–4 minutes. Add the warmed sugar to the pan and cook very gently over low heat, stirring the mixture carefully, until all the sugar has dissolved.

M AKING J AMS

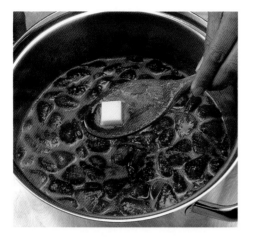

3 If desired, stir in the butter to reduce scum formation. Put a saucer to chill in the freezer.

WATCHPOINTS
- **Cloudy jam:** *The fruit was bruised or not clean. Discard.*
- **Crystallized, grainy jam:** *The jam was boiled before all the sugar had dissolved completely. To rectify, boil the jam, adding a little water or alcohol such as whiskey, or a liqueur, then put back into jars.*
- **Dark, runny jam:** *The jam was overboiled beyond the setting point.*
- **Jam that does not set or is syrupy:** *The jam was not boiled long enough (rectify by reboiling to reach setting point); there was insufficient pectin in the fruit (rectify by returning to a full boil, adding 3 tablespoons each of lemon juice and pectin extract or commercial liquid pectin, then boiling 1 minute more).*

- **Jam that ferments in storage:** *The jam was not boiled long enough. Fermented jams are harmless and can be reboiled until they reach setting point; reboiling may spoil the flavor and color of the jam.*
- **Hard, dry jam with poor color and flavor:** *The jam was boiled too long; it has been stored in a warm or damp place.*
- **Moldy jam:** *The jars were not sterilized, or were cold, damp or underfilled; if the jars were improperly sealed or processed, the jam may have been infected by mold spores in the air; the jam has been stored in a warm or damp place. Discard.*
- **Air pockets:** *The jam was too cool when it was poured into the jars.*
- **Fruit rises to top of jam:** *The jam was not left to stand before putting into jars.*

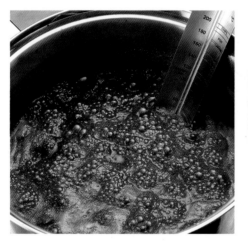 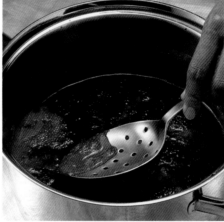 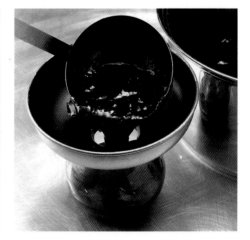

4 Raise the heat and boil the jam vigorously without stirring, until setting point is reached. This should take about 4 minutes (for recipes using ordinary sugar, test after 10–15 minutes). To test for set, remove the pan from the heat and drop a little jam onto the cold saucer. Push it gently with the tip of a teaspoon or your finger. If the surface wrinkles, setting point has been reached. Alternatively, test with a sugar thermometer (see page 17).

5 Using a slotted spoon, skim any scum from the surface of the jam. Leave to stand for 10–15 minutes before putting into jars, so that the fruit does not rise to the top but is evenly distributed throughout the jam when the jars are filled.

6 Ladle the jam into hot, clean, dry jars through a heatproof funnel, up to ½ inch from the top. Wipe jar rims and threads clean. Cover jars with dome metal caps, placing sealing compound-sides-down next to glass jar rims; screw the metal bands on tightly. Process in a simmering-water bath (185°F) for 10 minutes (see page 13). Transfer jars to a wire rack to cool. After 12 hours, test seals. Label sealed jars and store in a cool, dry, dark place.

Making Jellies

Jellies are often more versatile than jams, as they can be served with savory as well as sweet dishes. For sparkling, crystal-clear jellies, the fruit mixture must be strained through a special jelly bag (see page 10), which can take anywhere from 8 to 12 hours. If you are not concerned about clarity, the time can be reduced by using a sieve lined with a double thickness of cheesecloth and, if you are really pushed for time, by lightly squeezing the fruit in the sieve. The recipe below shows the basic method of jelly making, and also explains how you can incorporate herbs and other flavorings during the cooking process. Use it as a reference when making the jellies in this book.

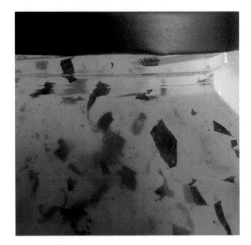

Orange and Tarragon Jelly

MAKES 4–4⅔ CUPS

3 pounds oranges, sliced
12 ounces lemons, sliced
¼ cup chopped fresh tarragon
warmed sugar (see page 7)

EQUIPMENT
• Sharp stainless steel kitchen knives
• Chopping board
• Measuring cup
• Scales
• Preserving pan or large nonaluminum saucepan
• Long-handled wooden spoon
• Jelly bag or large piece of fine cotton or enough cheesecloth to make a triple thickness
• Upturned stool or other means of supporting jelly bag
• Sugar thermometer (optional)
• Saucer and teaspoon
• Slotted spoon
• Funnel
• Suitable jars, lids or covers (see pages 10–11)

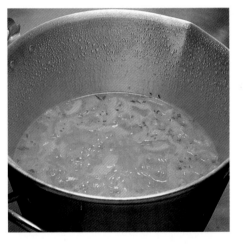

1 Chop the fruit slices and put them in a large saucepan with 2 quarts water and half the tarragon. Bring to a boil, then simmer gently, stirring occasionally with a wooden spoon to prevent sticking, for about 1¼ hours or until soft.

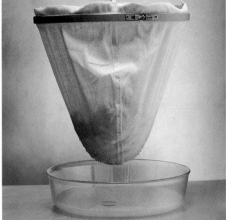

2 Scald the jelly bag – or cotton or cheesecloth, whichever you are using – by pouring boiling water through it. Tie the bag or cloth to the legs of an upturned stool and place a large nonmetallic or stainless steel bowl underneath the jelly bag. Pour the contents of the pan into the bag or cloth and leave to strain, undisturbed, in a cool place for 8–12 hours or until the liquid has stopped dripping through.

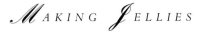

Making Jellies

3 Measure the juice collected in the bowl and pour it back into the rinsed-out pan. Add 2¼ cups warmed sugar for every 2½ cups juice. Heat gently, stirring, until the sugar has completely dissolved, then raise the heat and boil vigorously until the setting point is reached. Do not allow gas flames to rise up the sides of the pan. Stir the juice occasionally to make sure the jelly cooks evenly and to prevent it from burning.

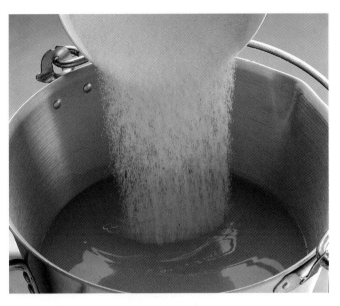

WATCHPOINTS
- **Cloudy jelly:** *The fruit was damaged or not clean; the jelly bag was not clean; the jelly bag was squeezed or pressed while the juice was being strained through it.*
- **Grainy, crystallized sugar:** *The strained juice was boiled before all the sugar had completely dissolved.*
- **Syrupy, dark jelly that will not set:** *The jelly was overboiled beyond setting point.*
- **Watery jelly that will not set:** *The jelly was not boiled long enough; rectify by reboiling the jelly.*
- **Moldy jelly:** *The jars were cold or damp or they were underfilled; the jelly has not been properly stored in a cool, dark, dry place. Discard.*

See also Making Jams (pages 14–15)

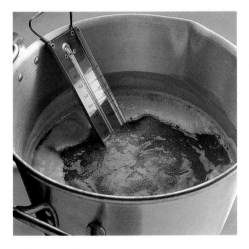

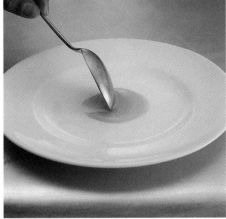

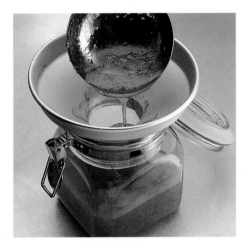

4 A sugar thermometer lets you know how boiling is proceeding: Clip it onto the side of the pan if you can, or hold it for a short while well down in the boiling jelly but away from the bottom of the pan. Jellies set best at a temperature of 8 degrees higher than the boiling point of water in your area. Most jellies set at 221°F, but some fruits may need a degree higher or lower, so double check with a saucer test.

5 To test for set, chill a saucer in the freezer before starting the second boiling. When ready to test, remove the pan from the heat and drop a little jelly onto the cold saucer. Push it gently with the tip of a teaspoon or your finger. If the surface wrinkles, setting point has been reached. With the pan still off the heat, skim off any scum from the surface of the jelly with a slotted spoon. Stir in the remaining tarragon. Let the jelly stand for 10–15 minutes.

6 Ladle the jelly into hot, clean, dry jars through a heatproof funnel, up to ½ inch from the top. Wipe jar rims and threads clean. Cover jars with dome metal caps, placing sealing compound-sides-down next to glass jar rims; screw the metal bands on tightly. Process in a simmering-water bath (185°F) for 10 minutes (see page 13). Transfer jars to a wire rack to cool. After 12 hours, test seals. Label sealed jars and store in a cool, dry, dark place.

Making Marmalades

Marmalades are made in much the same way as jams. They can be chunky, thin-cut, or fine-shred, depending on how the peel is prepared. The initial cooking time is often long because citrus peels are thicker than fruit skins, so they take longer to soften. Bitter Seville oranges are, of course, the king of the marmalade fruits. They appear only briefly from November through January; the best places to look for them are Hispanic grocery stores, Latin American markets and specialty produce stores. Buy fairly large amounts; what you don't use right away can be put into plastic bags and frozen to use later (pectin deteriorates with time, so add 1 extra orange per pound).

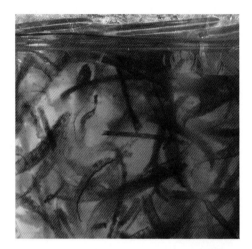

Seville Orange Marmalade

MAKES ABOUT 6⅔ CUPS

**1½ pounds Seville oranges
juice of 1 large lemon
7 cups sugar**

EQUIPMENT
- Sharp stainless steel kitchen knives
- Chopping board
- Lemon juicer
- Small piece of cheesecloth
- Kitchen string
- Preserving pan or very large nonaluminum saucepan
- Slotted spoon
- Wooden spoon
- Saucer and teaspoon
- Sugar thermometer (optional)
- Funnel
- Suitable jars, lids or covers (see pages 10–11)

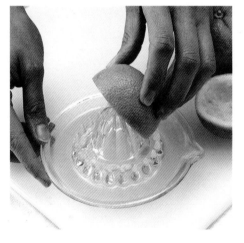

1 Halve the oranges. Squeeze out all the juice, reserving the seeds and membrane that comes away during squeezing.

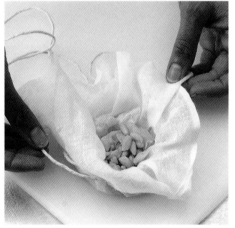

2 Place the seeds and membrane on a piece of cheesecloth. Tie into a bag with a long length of string.

*M*AKING *M*ARMALADES

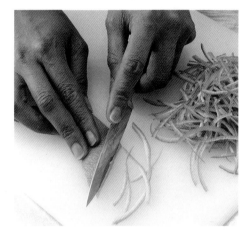

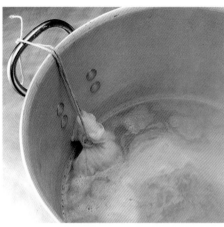

- **Tough peel:** *The peel was not cooked long enough before the sugar was added.*
- **Peel rises to top of jar:** *The marmalade was not left to stand for 10–15 minutes before being put into jars.*
- **Shrinkage on storage:** *The marmalade was not covered correctly; the marmalade was not processed properly in the water bath; the marmalade has not been kept in a cool, dark, dry place. Discard.*

See also Making Jams (pages 14–15)

3 Slice the orange peel as required and put into a saucepan with the orange and lemon juices and 6 cups water.

4 Tie the string to the pan handle so the bag is suspended in the mixture. Bring to a boil, then simmer for 1–1½ hours.

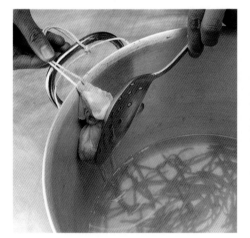

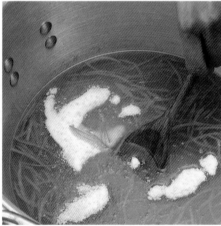

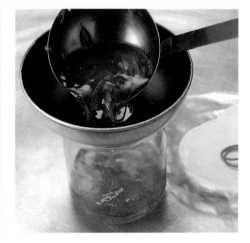

5 At the end of the boiling time, the peel should be soft and the liquid reduced by half. Scoop out the cheesecloth bag with a slotted spoon and squeeze it firmly against the side of the pan so that the juice runs back into the pan. Discard the bag.
  Chill a saucer for testing for a set.

6 Using a wooden spoon, stir the sugar into the marmalade over low heat until the sugar is dissolved. Raise the heat and boil vigorously for 10–15 minutes, stirring as necessary, until setting point has been reached. To test for set, remove the pan from the heat and drop a little marmalade onto the cold saucer. Push it gently with the tip of a teaspoon or your finger. If the surface wrinkles, setting point has been reached. Alternatively, use a sugar thermometer (see page 17).

7 Stir the marmalade and ladle into hot, clean, dry jars through a heatproof funnel, up to ½ inch from the top. Wipe jar rims and threads clean. Cover jars with dome metal caps, placing sealing compound-sides-down next to glass jar rims; screw the metal bands on tightly. Process in a simmering-water bath (185°F) for 10 minutes (see page 13). Transfer jars to a wire rack to cool. After 12 hours, test seals. Label sealed jars and store them in a cool, dry, dark place.

Making Candied Fruits

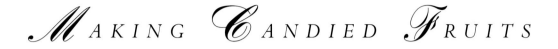

Good candied, crystallized, and glacé fruit is expensive to buy but can be prepared at home without much difficulty. The process may seem rather lengthy, but the results are worth the effort. Use firm, ripe, unbruised fruit.

For plums, apricots, and kumquats: Prick all over with a large embroidery needle so that the syrup will penetrate evenly and right through to the center. For cherries: Remove the pits using a cherry pitter. For citrus fruits (except kumquats): Peel and divide into segments, removing all the skin and pith. For pears, apples, and peaches: Peel, then halve or thickly slice. For pineapple: Remove the skin, eyes, and core; cut into chunks or rings.

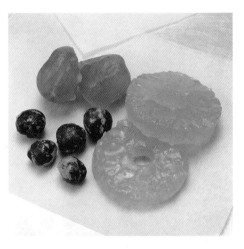

Candied fruit: For each 1 pound fruit, you will need 3½ cups sugar
Crystallized fruit: For each 1 pound candied fruit, you will need about 1¼ cups superfine sugar
Glacé fruit: For each 1 pound candied fruit, you will need 2¼ cups (1 pound) sugar

EQUIPMENT
For candied fruit:
• Large embroidery needle, cherry pitter, and sharp kitchen knives
• Kitchen scales
• 2 saucepans
• Slotted spoon and wooden spoon
• Wire basket to fit inside second saucepan
• Measuring cup
• Wire rack
• Aluminum foil
For crystallized fruit, you also need:
• Skewer
• Small bowl
• Baking tray
For glacé fruit, you also need:
• 2 saucepans (1 large and 1 small)
• Cup or small bowl
• Skewer
Plus suitable boxes or containers, waxed paper

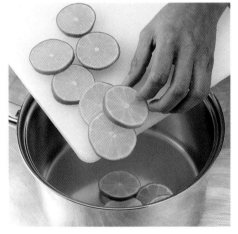

1 Weigh the fruit after it has been prepared (see above). Put the fruit in a large saucepan, add just enough boiling water to cover, then simmer gently, covered, until tender – soft fruits take only 2–3 minutes; firm ones, such as apricots, 10–15 minutes. Using a slotted spoon, transfer the fruit to a wire basket placed inside another saucepan.

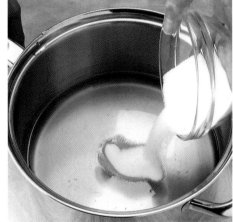

2 For every 1 pound of prepared fruit, measure out 1¼ cups of the cooking water and ¾ cup plus 2 tablespoons sugar. Combine in a saucepan and gently heat, stirring with a wooden spoon, until the sugar has dissolved. Raise the heat and bring the liquid to a boil.

*M*AKING *C*ANDIED *F*RUITS

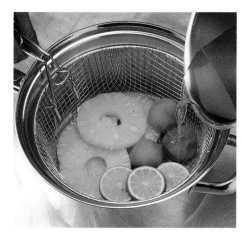

3 Pour the hot syrup over the fruit, cover, and leave for 1 day in a cool place. The next day, lift out the basket with the fruit.

4 Add another ⅓ cup sugar to the syrup and dissolve over low heat, stirring. Raise the heat, bring to a boil, then remove from the heat and lower the fruit into the pan once more. Cover and leave in a cool place for 1 day. Repeat this step daily for the next 5 days, so that the syrup gradually becomes more concentrated.

5 Lift the basket containing the fruit from the saucepan, add 7 tablespoons sugar to the syrup, and heat gently, stirring, until the sugar has dissolved. Lower the fruit back into the pan and simmer gently for 3–4 minutes. Remove from the heat, cover, and leave in a cool place for 2 days. Repeat this step once more, but leave the fruit to stand for 4 days or up to 2 weeks.

6 Lift the wire basket containing the fruit from the sugar syrup for the last time and, using a pair of tongs, transfer each piece of fruit to a wire rack placed over a tray to dry. Protect the fruit from dust by placing a dome of aluminum foil over the wire rack, making sure that it does not touch the surface of the fruit. Leave the fruit in a warm, dry place for 2–3 days, turning each piece over two or three times, until it is completely dry.

Using a pair of tongs, carefully pack the fruit into attractive boxes or other containers, placing waxed paper between each layer. If you have used an assortment of fruits, you can either layer them according to type or mix the fruit together for an attractive, colorful presentation.

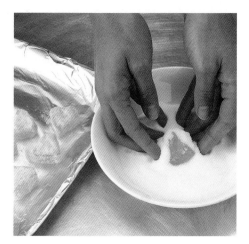

Crystallized Fruit

To make crystallized fruits, you have to candy them first (see above). Fill a small bowl with superfine sugar and bring a saucepan of water to a boil. Spear each piece of completely dry candied fruit with a skewer and quickly dip it in the boiling water. Allow any excess moisture to drain off, then roll the fruit in the superfine sugar. Transfer to a foil-lined tray and leave to dry.

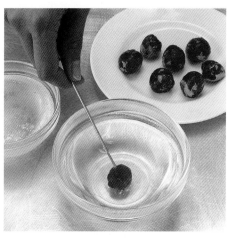

Glacé Fruit

Candied fruits are also the starting point for glacé fruits. Heat ⅔ cup water with the sugar (see page 20) and stir until the sugar has dissolved. Boil for 1 minute. Pour a little hot syrup into a warm bowl. Cover the syrup in the pan and place in a saucepan of simmering water to keep warm. Spear each piece of fruit with a skewer, dip into boiling water for 20 seconds, then dip into the syrup.

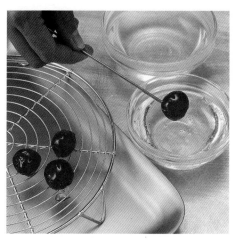

As each piece of fruit is ready, transfer it to a wire rack placed over a tray. As the syrup in the cup becomes cloudy, discard it and add fresh hot syrup.

Cover the fruit with a dome of aluminum foil. Leave to dry in a warm place for 2–3 days, turning a few times.

WATCHPOINTS
• **Shapeless or tough fruit:** *The soft fruit was cooked too long at the beginning.*

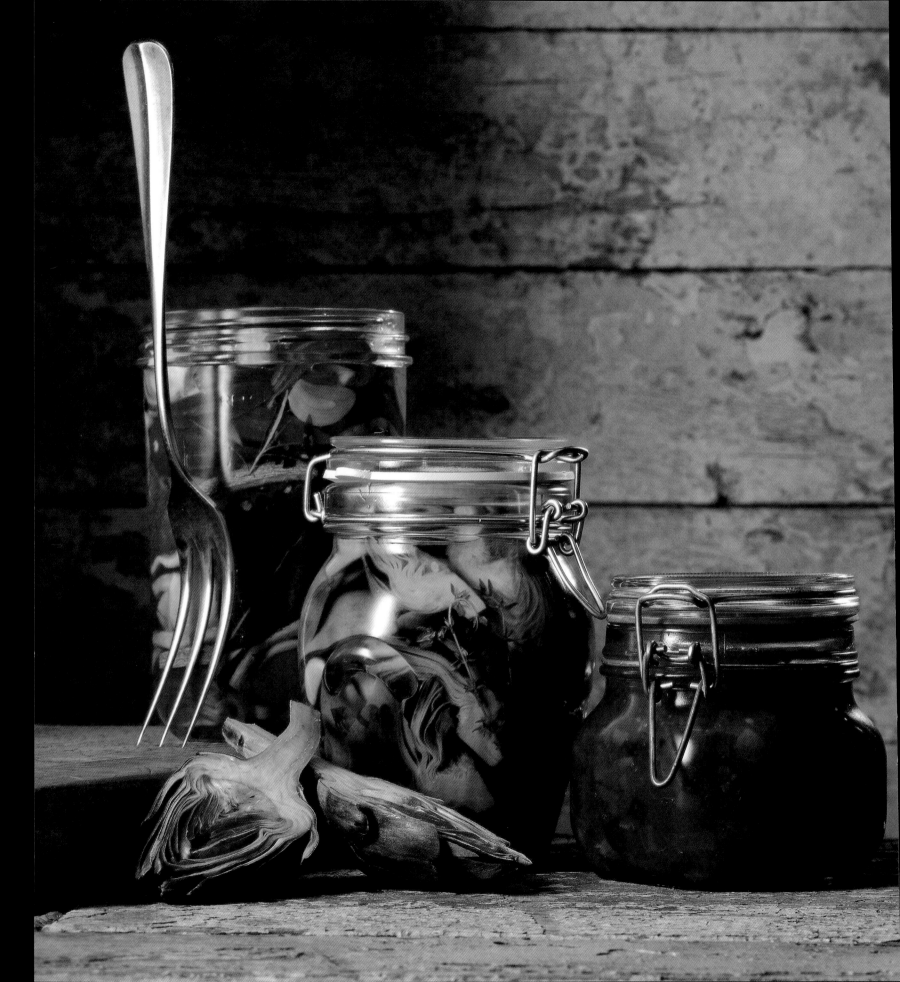

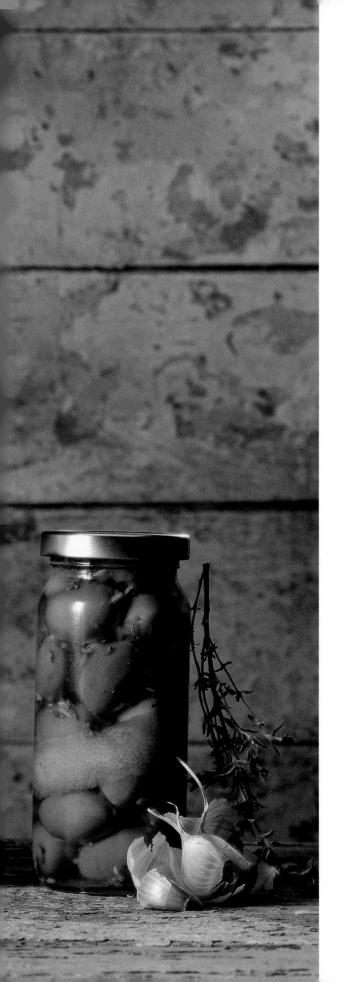

𝒱EGETABLES

This chapter contains an enormous variety of vegetable preserves, from modest Pickled Baby Beets (see page 26) to the more upmarket Artichokes in Oil (see page 24), Angel's Hair (see page 27), and fashionable Roasted Red Peppers in Oil (see page 32), which come into their own in a delicious Fettuccine with Smoked Trout, Basil, and Roasted Red Peppers (see page 33). Preserved vegetables are real pantry stalwarts. With this imaginative and mouthwatering selection of recipes, you need never be at a loss for a snack, an appetizer, a vegetable accompaniment, or something unusual to boost a main course or liven up a salad, picnic, or buffet.

Left, from left to right: Italian Garden Pickle, Artichokes in Oil, Ratatouille Chutney, and Spiced Green Olives.

Artichokes in Oil

If you are able to find very small artichokes, preserve them whole, as the Italians do.

MAKES 4½ CUPS

3 pounds artichokes
½ lemon
1 quart white wine vinegar
2¼ cups dry white wine
3 sprigs of fresh thyme
1 small sprig of fresh rosemary
6 garlic cloves
about 3½ cups olive oil
2 dried red chilies (optional)

Snap the stems from the artichokes and trim away the outer leaves. Trim the tops of the leaves, then cut the artichokes into halves or quarters. Cut out the hairy chokes. Drop the artichokes into a bowl of water acidulated with a good squeeze of lemon juice.

Combine the vinegar, wine, 2 sprigs of thyme, and the rosemary in a large saucepan, then bring to a boil.

Tie the garlic in a square of cheesecloth and add to the pan for several seconds. Fish out and reserve the bag.

Add the artichokes to the pan and cook for about 20 minutes or until tender. Drain them and leave to dry on paper towels.

Pour a thin layer of oil into a preserving jar. Using a spoon, add a layer of artichokes; pack them in well so that no air is trapped. Pour in more oil, add a garlic clove and a little crumbled chili if using, then repeat the layering. Insert the remaining thyme sprig along the side of the jar when it is partly filled. Cover the artichokes with oil before sealing and processing the jar (see pages 12–13). Store in a cool, dark, dry place for at least 2 months before eating.

Serving Suggestion
Toss with chopped parsley, a squeeze of lemon juice, black pepper, chopped dried red chili, and a little olive oil.

Artichoke and Mushroom Pizza

Use Artichokes in Oil and mushrooms to transform a store-bought pizza base.

SERVES 2

4 ounces oyster mushrooms, sliced
2–3 tablespoons oil from Artichokes in Oil (see left)
1–1½ cups Artichokes in Oil (see left)
squeeze of lemon juice
10-inch prepared pizza base
3–4 ounces fontina cheese, grated
sea salt and freshly ground black pepper
chopped fresh thyme for sprinkling

Preheat the oven to 425°F.

Sauté the mushrooms in a little of the artichoke oil, then toss them together with the artichokes.

Mix a squeeze of lemon juice with the remaining artichoke oil and brush over the pizza base. Distribute the artichokes and mushrooms evenly over the base, then scatter the cheese over the top. Bake the pizza for about 20 minutes or according to package instructions. Sprinkle with thyme and serve.

Below: Artichoke and Mushroom Pizza. You can add more artichokes and mushrooms for an extra-generous topping.

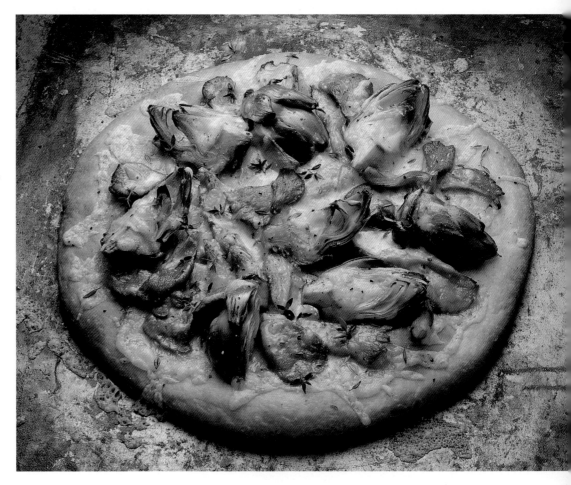

*E*GGPLANTS

Eggplant and Pepper Pickle

MAKES ABOUT 3⅓ CUPS

1 pound eggplants
sea salt
4 large red bell peppers or 2 red and 2 yellow peppers
1¼ cups white wine vinegar
1–2 garlic cloves, cut into slivers
about 1¼ cups olive oil
6 anchovy fillets, drained
2–3 teaspoons capers, preferably salt-packed, drained
1 teaspoon black peppercorns
several fresh basil leaves

Preheat the broiler to high. Cut the eggplants in half lengthwise, then cut into ¼-inch slices. Layer the slices in a nonmetallic colander, sprinkling each layer with salt. Leave to drain for 2–3 hours.

Meanwhile, broil the peppers until the skins are charred and blistered. Leave until they are cool enough to handle, then peel them. Discard the cores and seeds and cut the flesh into ¼-inch strips.

Rinse the eggplant slices well under running cold water, then drain and dry them thoroughly on paper towels.

Bring the vinegar and ⅔ cup water to a boil in a large saucepan; add the eggplant and garlic and blanch for 1 minute. Drain.

Pour a little oil into a warm, clean, dry 1-quart jar, then layer the eggplant, garlic, and peppers in the jar, adding an anchovy fillet, 2 or 3 capers, 1 or 2 peppercorns, and a basil leaf here and there. Add more oil between the layers. Cover completely with olive oil and rotate the jar to make sure all the air is expelled, then cover, seal, and process (see pages 12–13). Store in a cool, dark, dry place for 1 month before eating.

Middle Eastern Stuffed Eggplants in Oil

Pickled vegetables are very popular in the Middle East. Many families still prepare large glass jars (*martabans*) filled with vegetables, and colorful displays are a common sight in shop windows.

MAKES 3¾ CUPS

2 pounds small eggplants
sea salt
4 garlic cloves, finely chopped
1–2 small dried red chilies, seeded and finely chopped
leaves from several sprigs of fresh cilantro or parsley
1–1¼ cups olive oil

Cut off the stem ends of the eggplants. Make a small slit in the middle of each eggplant, then place them in a large pan of salted water and poach over low heat for about 20 minutes or until they are tender; keep the eggplants submerged with a heavy lid that will fit inside the pan.

Drain the eggplants and leave them until they are cool enough to handle, then squeeze them to remove the juices.

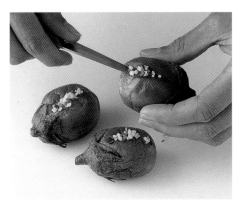

Stuffing eggplant: Use a sharp knife to ease the chili mixture into each eggplant for Middle Eastern Stuffed Eggplants in Oil.

Mix together the garlic, chilies, cilantro or parsley, and a pinch of salt.

Enlarge the slit in each eggplant and insert some of the chili mixture (see below).

Pack the eggplants into a clean, dry 1-quart jar and pour in oil to cover. Cover, seal, and process (see pages 12–13). Store in a cool, dark, dry place for 2–4 weeks before opening.

Eggplant, Okra, and Cilantro Relish

Choose small, unblemished, completely green okra for this fragrant relish.

MAKES ABOUT 4 CUPS

1 pound eggplants, cut into thick chunks
4 teaspoons sea salt
1 large onion, coarsely chopped
2 garlic cloves, crushed
2 celery stalks, coarsely chopped
8 ounces small okra, sliced
2 tablespoons tomato purée
1–2 tablespoons curry powder, to taste
2 teaspoons ground allspice
1 teaspoon ground ginger
10 tablespoons soft brown sugar
5 cups white wine vinegar
2 tablespoons chopped fresh cilantro

Layer the eggplants and salt in a nonmetallic colander. Leave to drain overnight.

Dry but do not rinse the eggplants, then put into a pan with the other ingredients except the cilantro. Simmer for 30 minutes, stir in the cilantro, then pack into warm, clean, dry jars. Cover with acid-proof lids, seal, and process (see pages 12–13). Store the relish in a cool, dark, dry place for 2–4 weeks before eating.

Serving Suggestion
Serve as an accompaniment to Indian food.

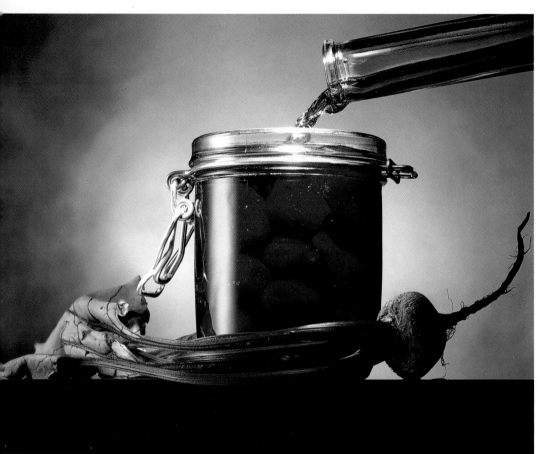

Pickled Baby Beets

Choose baby beets with unbruised and blemish-free skins. Do not peel them until after they have been cooked; otherwise, the color will bleed. Most pickles are bottled cold, but because of the size of the beets in this recipe, the jars are filled when the ingredients are still hot.

MAKES ABOUT 2⅔ CUPS

2 pounds baby beets, left whole
1–1½ teaspoons sugar
2 teaspoons salt
2½ cups Spiced Vinegar (see page 139), made with red wine vinegar
allspice berries

Cook the beets in boiling water for 30–40 minutes or until tender. Drain and rinse the beets under cold running water and leave until cool enough to handle.

Meanwhile, gently heat the sugar and salt in the spiced vinegar until dissolved, stirring frequently, then bring to a boil. Remove from the heat and set aside to cool.

When the beets are cool enough to handle, peel them and pack them into warm, clean, dry jars. Add 2 allspice berries to each jar. Pour in the vinegar and rotate the jars to expel any air, then cover with acid-proof lids, seal, and process (see pages 12–13). Store in a cool, dark, dry place for at least 1 month before eating.

Variation: If baby beets are not available, wrap larger beets in foil and bake at 350°F for 2–3 hours, depending on size. Peel and thinly slice the beets when they are cool, then pack them into warm, clean, dry jars. Cover with the spiced vinegar, adding 2 teaspoons salt for every 2½ cups vinegar; omit the sugar.

Beet and Horseradish Relish

Horseradish, beets, and apples make a fruity relish with a piquant flavor. Use a food processor rather than an ordinary grater to grate the horseradish to protect yourself against eye-watering fumes.

MAKES ABOUT 4 CUPS

1 pound raw beets
2 ounces horseradish, grated
4 ounces onion, chopped
8 ounces cooking apples, peeled, cored, and chopped
⅔ cup sugar
1½ cups cider vinegar

Above: Pickled Baby Beets are delicious eaten with cold roast meats.

Peel the beets, then grate coarsely into a large saucepan. Add the remaining ingredients and heat gently, stirring, until the sugar has dissolved. Slowly bring to a boil and continue to boil gently for about 1¼ hours, stirring occasionally, until the vegetables and apples are tender and the relish well reduced. Ladle into warm, clean, dry jars. Cover with acid-proof lids, seal, and process (see pages 12–13). Store in a cool, dark, dry place for 4–6 weeks before eating.

Serving Suggestion
This relish will perk up cold roast beef or pork, steaks, and cheese.

Pickled Red Cabbage with Orange

Oranges and raisins make a fruity, mildly flavored pickled cabbage.

MAKES ABOUT 5⅓ CUPS

1 red cabbage, about 2 pounds, halved, cored, and shredded
2 tablespoons sea salt
2½ cups Spiced Vinegar (see page 139), made with red wine vinegar
1 large onion, thinly sliced
⅓ cup raisins
juice and finely grated zest of 2 large oranges
1 tablespoon brown sugar

Put the cabbage into a large nonmetallic bowl. Stir in the salt and leave for 8 hours.

Meanwhile, bring the vinegar with its spices and bay leaf to a boil, then remove from the heat, cover, and leave to cool.

Rinse the cabbage thoroughly, then drain and dry. Pack into warm, clean, dry jars.

Put the spiced vinegar, onion, raisins, orange juice, zest, and sugar into a pan. Heat gently, stirring, until the sugar has dissolved, then bring to a boil. Pour over the cabbage, shaking the jars gently to make sure it is well distributed. Cover with acid-proof lids, seal, and process (see pages 12–13). Store in a cool, dark, dry place for at least 1 month before eating.

Serving Suggestion
Serve with cold duck or game, especially venison and squab.

Right: Pickled Red Cabbage with Orange has a delicious fruity tang and is less harshly flavored than most ordinary red cabbage preserves.

Angel's Hair

"Angel's hair" is a rather fanciful name for this eye-catching carrot jam.

MAKES ABOUT 1⅓ CUPS

about 10 ounces carrots, scraped and grated to yield about 1½ cups
1¼ cups sugar
1 large lemon
3 cardamom pods, split

Put the carrots and sugar into a saucepan.

Cut the lemon peel into thin strips, squeeze the juice from the lemon, then put both into the pan with the cardamom pods.

Heat gently, stirring, until the sugar has dissolved, then boil for 10 minutes or until very thick. Skim with a slotted spoon.

Spoon the jam into warm, clean, dry jars. Cover, seal, and process (see pages 12–13). The jam is now ready to eat. Store in a cool, dark, dry place for up to 1 year.

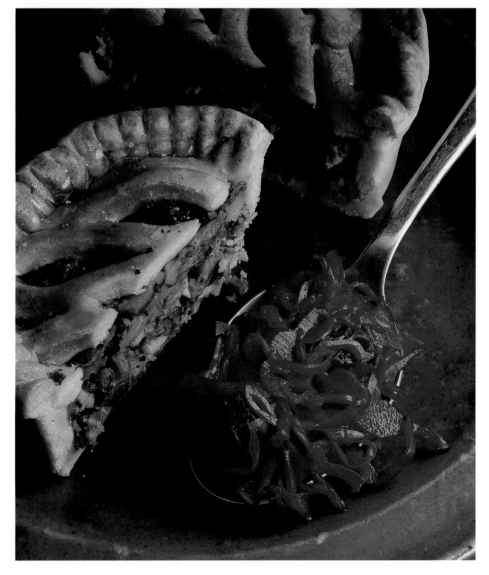

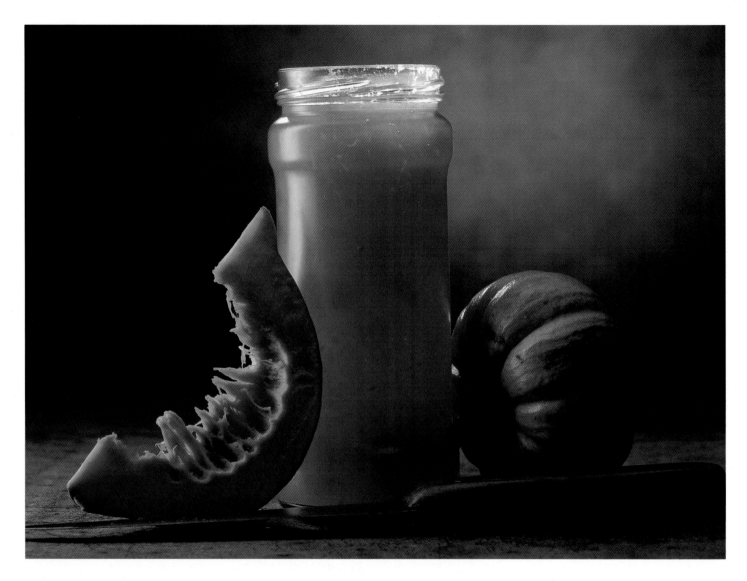

Pumpkin Preserve

This attractive orange preserve is spiced with ginger. Country markets are often the best places to buy pumpkins.

1 pumpkin, sliced, peeled, seeds and strings discarded, and diced
For each 1 pound prepared pumpkin flesh:
2¼ cups sugar
1 ounce fresh ginger, grated
juice of ½ lemon

Steam the pumpkin for about 20 minutes or until tender.

Stir the pumpkin, sugar, ginger, and lemon juice together in a nonmetallic bowl. Cover and leave in a cool place for 24 hours.

Transfer the pumpkin mixture to a large heavy-based saucepan and stir over low heat until the sugar has dissolved. Then boil vigorously for about 15 minutes, stirring if necessary, until it is thick and translucent.

Ladle into warm, clean, dry jars. Cover, seal, and process (see pages 12–13).

Above: Bright orange Pumpkin Preserve is ideal for making in the fall, then serving at Thanksgiving or Christmas.

Leave the jars to cool, then store the preserve in a cool, dark, dry place for at least 1 month before eating.

Serving Suggestion
Try this in place of jam or marmalade for breakfast or with fresh ricotta cheese or thick yogurt for a quick dessert.

Gherkins, Turnips, and Olives

Pickled Gherkins

Gherkins, also known by the French name of *cornichons*, are a variety of small cucumber about 1½–2 inches long. Specially grown for pickling, gherkins can be found at the market from about the end of June through September.

MAKES 3 CUPS

1 pound small firm gherkins
⅔ cup salt
2 cloves
1 teaspoon black peppercorns
1 teaspoon allspice berries
1 blade of mace
2½ cups white wine vinegar

Put the gherkins in a nonmetallic bowl. Stir the salt into 2½ cups of water until dissolved, then pour over the gherkins and stir. Cover and leave in a cool, dark, dry place for 3 days.

Drain the gherkins, then rinse and dry them thoroughly. Put into a large, warm, dry, heatproof jar.

Put the spices and vinegar into a saucepan, bring to a boil, and boil for 10 minutes. Pour over the gherkins, cover tightly and leave in a warm place for 24 hours.

Drain the vinegar from the jar into a saucepan. Bring to a boil, then pour back over the gherkins. Cover tightly again and leave in a cool place for another 24 hours. The gherkins should now be a strong, vivid green color. If this is not the case, repeat the process as many times as necessary until the correct color has been achieved.

Pack the gherkins into warm, clean, dry jars. Bring the vinegar to a boil once more and pour into the jars to cover the gherkins. Cover with acid-proof lids, seal, and process (see pages 12–13). Store in a cool, dark, dry place for 2 weeks before eating.

Serving Suggestion
Eat with pâtés or hard cheeses.

Dill Pickled Gherkins

Dill seeds and onions give this basic pickled gherkin recipe an extra herby flavor.

MAKES ABOUT 3 CUPS

2¼ pounds small firm gherkins
2¾ cups sea salt
3 cups white wine vinegar
2 teaspoons dill seeds
3½ ounces very small pickling onions
2 garlic cloves

Put the gherkins in a nonmetallic bowl, sprinkle with the salt, and leave to stand in a cool place for about 24 hours.

Drain the gherkins, rinse thoroughly, then drain and dry well on paper towels. Return to the rinsed and dried bowl.

Bring the vinegar to a boil, then simmer for 5 minutes. Pour over the gherkins, cover the bowl, and leave in the refrigerator for 1 day. Drain off the vinegar into a saucepan, bring it to a boil again, then leave to cool completely.

Pack the gherkins, dill seeds, onions, and garlic into a jar. Pour in vinegar to cover and rotate the jar to expel any air. Cover the jar with an acid-proof lid, seal, and process (see pages 12–13). Store in a cool, dark, dry place for at least 2 months before using.

Serving Suggestion
Serve with spicy sausages or salami.

Pickled Turnips

This pickle has a delicate sweet sharpness and light crispness that are very appealing.

MAKES ABOUT 3⅔ CUPS

¼ cup sea salt
1 cup white wine vinegar
2 pounds small turnips, peeled and halved
1 small raw beet, peeled and sliced

2–4 garlic cloves (optional)
a few celery leaves

Gently heat 2 cups water with the salt, stirring. Bring to a boil, remove from the heat, add the vinegar, and leave to cool.

Layer the turnips, beet slices, garlic if using, and celery leaves in a clean, dry jar. Pour in the cooled brine to completely cover. Rotate the jar to expel any air. Hold the turnips down with crumpled waxed paper placed at the top of the jar. Seal the jar tightly and process (see pages 12–13) and leave on a sunny windowsill or in a warm place for about 2 weeks before eating.

Unopened jars will keep for 3 months, but once opened, they should be refrigerated.

Spiced Green Olives

Here's a good way of livening up olives that are not the best quality. The oil can be used for salad dressings or in cooking.

MAKES 1⅓ CUPS

8 ounces green olives packed in brine, rinsed
1 tablespoon fennel seeds, lightly crushed
4 large garlic cloves, crushed
long strip of lemon zest
4 sprigs of fresh thyme
about ¾ cup olive oil

Using a meat mallet or hammer, lightly tap the olives to split them, but leave the pits intact. Alternatively, make a cut in each olive with a knife. Dry the olives on paper towels.

Pack the olives into a clean, dry jar along with the fennel seeds, garlic, lemon zest, and sprigs of thyme.

Pour in enough oil to cover the olives completely, rotating the jar to expel any air. Cover, seal, and process (see pages 12–13). Store in a cool, dark, dry place for 2 weeks before eating, shaking the jar occasionally.

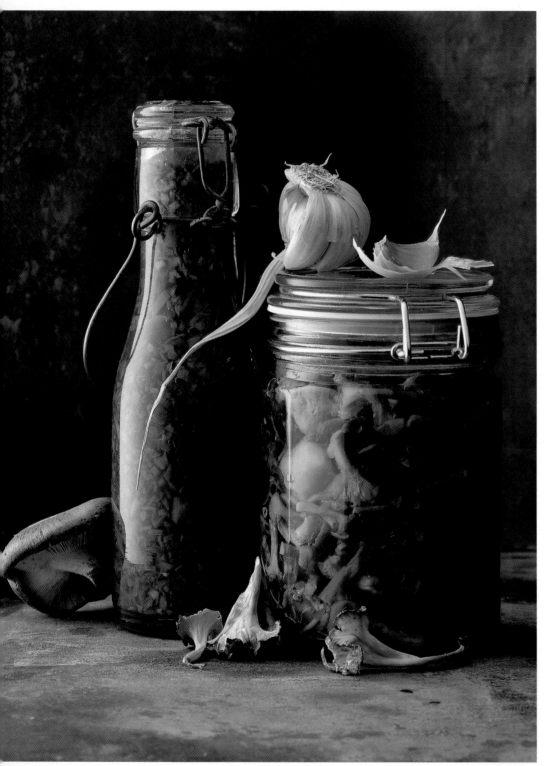

Mushrooms in Oil

MAKES ABOUT 2 QUARTS

½ onion, finely chopped
½ small red bell pepper, cored, seeded, and finely chopped
2 garlic cloves, crushed
about ¾ cup olive oil
1¾ cups white wine vinegar
few sprigs of fresh parsley
few sprigs of fresh thyme
1 sprig of fresh rosemary
3 fresh bay leaves
5 coriander seeds, crushed
10 black peppercorns, crushed
2 pounds mushrooms

Gently sauté the onion, pepper, and garlic in a little of the oil in a large saucepan until softened but not colored. Add the vinegar, herbs, coriander seeds, peppercorns, and 1⅔ cups water. Bring to a boil, then continue boiling, uncovered, for 10 minutes.

Put the mushrooms in a large nonmetallic bowl and pour the contents of the saucepan over them. Submerge the mushrooms with a plate and leave for 12 hours; stir occasionally. Drain off the liquid, then transfer the mushrooms, herbs, and vegetables to paper towels to dry.

Using a slotted spoon, pack the herbs and vegetables into a clean, dry jar. Slowly pour in enough olive oil to cover completely, pressing down on the mushrooms to expel air. Rotate the jar to release any air bubbles, then cover, seal, and process (see pages 12–13). Store in a cool, dark, dry place for at least 3–4 weeks before eating.

Serving Suggestion

Add to chicken cooked in wine, then stir in a little heavy cream or crème fraîche to finish. Use the mushroom oil to sauté the chicken.

Far left and left: Mushroom Ketchup and Mushrooms in Oil. Use white mushrooms or try shiitake and oyster mushrooms.

Mushrooms, Onions, and Shallots

Mushroom Ketchup

MAKES ABOUT 2 CUPS

2 pounds mushrooms, finely chopped
¼ teaspoon ground cloves
½ teaspoon each ground mace and allspice
2 anchovy fillets, chopped
1¼ cups ruby port
sea salt and plenty of freshly ground
   black pepper

Bring all the ingredients and 5 tablespoons water to a slow boil in a large saucepan. Simmer for 10 minutes, stirring occasionally, until the mixture starts to thicken.

   Pour the mixture into a warm, clean, dry jar, then cover loosely and leave to cool. Seal and process the jar (see pages 12–13) and store in a cool, dark, dry place for at least 10 days before using.

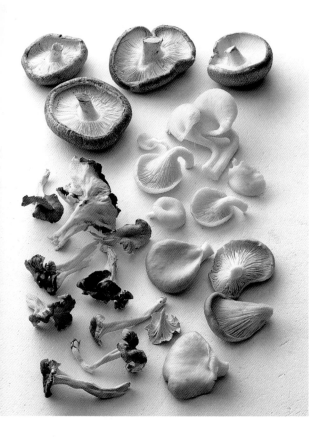

Savory Red Onion Relish

The fruity black currant flavor of Crème de Cassis gives the onions in this recipe a delicious, rich sweetness.

MAKES ABOUT 2⅔ CUPS

1½ pounds large red onions, thinly sliced
2 tablespoons olive oil
sea salt and freshly ground black pepper
6 tablespoons granulated sugar
1 cup red wine
4 tablespoons sherry vinegar
2 tablespoons Crème de Cassis (see page 87)
¼ teaspoon ground allspice

Cook the onions in the oil in a large skillet or a saucepan over very low heat until they are soft. Sprinkle with salt and pepper, stir in the sugar, cover, and cook for 10 minutes, stirring occasionally.

   Stir in the wine, sherry vinegar, crème de cassis, and allspice, then raise the heat and simmer, stirring frequently, for about 30 minutes or until thick.

   Ladle into warm, clean, dry jars. Cover with acid-proof lids, seal, and process (see pages 12–13). Store in a cool, dark, dry place for 2 or 3 days before eating.

Serving Suggestion
Serve hot or cold with broiled meats or poultry, homemade sausages, game terrine, or *pâté en croûte*; serve cold with a large wedge of mature Vermont Cheddar cheese, and crusty bread.

Left, clockwise from top left: shiitake, yellow oyster, oyster, and chanterelle mushrooms.

Shallot Confiture

This *confiture* is made over a number of days to give the shallots a silky character.

MAKES ABOUT 3⅓ CUPS

1½ pounds shallots, peeled, root ends intact
scant 1 cup sea salt
1 quart cider vinegar
2¼ cups sugar
1½ teaspoons whole cloves
2 cardamom pods, crushed
1½ teaspoons caraway seeds
1 long strip of lemon zest
1 cinnamon stick
2–4 dried red chilies, crushed
good pinch of ground chili

Put the shallots in a nonmetallic bowl, sprinkle with the salt, and add enough water to cover, stirring carefully to dissolve the salt. Put a plate on the shallots to submerge them, then leave for 1 day in a cool place.

   Drain and rinse the shallots thoroughly and dry on paper towels. Pour the vinegar into a large saucepan and stir in the sugar. Place the spices, except the ground chili, on a square of cheesecloth and tie into a bag. Add to the pan with the ground chili and heat gently, stirring, until the sugar has dissolved. Raise the heat and boil fairly vigorously for 10 minutes. Skim the surface scum with a slotted spoon.

   Add the shallots and simmer very gently for 15 minutes. Remove the pan from the heat, cover, and leave overnight.

   The next day, slowly bring the shallots to a boil, then simmer gently for another 15 minutes. Remove from the heat, cover, and leave overnight. The next day, slowly bring the shallots to a boil once more, then simmer gently until they are golden brown and translucent. Pack into warm, clean, dry jars, taking care not to trap any air pockets. Cover with acid-proof lids, seal, and process (see pages 12–13). Store in a cool, dark, dry place for 2 months before eating.

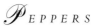
Pickled Red Peppers

Although it may seem that all red bell peppers are alike, there are a number of varieties available. You can also include some yellow bell peppers in this recipe, but I don't think green bell peppers work as well. Whichever you use, choose plump, fleshy ones.

MAKES ABOUT 1 QUART

4 large fleshy bell peppers, cored, seeded, and
   cut into strips
1 small red onion, finely chopped
sea salt
6–8 sun-dried tomatoes
about 3 small bay leaves
about 1½ cups white wine vinegar

Layer the peppers and onion alternately in a nonmetallic bowl, sprinkling each layer generously with salt. Cover with a plate to press the vegetables lightly and leave in a cool place for 24 hours, stirring gently from time to time.

Place the sun-dried tomatoes in a heatproof bowl, pour boiling water over them, and leave to soak for 5 minutes. Drain, dry on paper towels, then cut into thin strips.

Rinse the peppers and onion under cold running water, drain, and dry thoroughly on paper towels. Mix the peppers, onion, and tomatoes in a bowl, then pack into a clean, dry jar, adding the bay leaves. Pour in the vinegar to cover, rotating the jar to expel any air. Cover with an acid-proof lid, seal, and process (see pages 12–13). Store the pickled peppers in a cool, dark, dry place for 2 months before eating.

Serving Suggestion
Drain well and serve as a light first course sprinkled with virgin olive oil. Add some black olives, preferably oil-cured, strips of anchovy, and a sprinkling of parsley and serve as a simple first course or part of an *antipasto misto.* The peppers also go well with grilled or broiled chicken and fish.

Red Pepper Relish

This richly flavored relish goes well with hot, simply cooked meat and poultry, as well as with cold meats.

MAKES ABOUT 2 CUPS

2 plump red bell peppers, cored, seeded,
   and chopped
2 plump yellow bell peppers, cored, seeded,
   and chopped
1 large onion, chopped
3 plump garlic cloves, thinly sliced
2 dried red chilies, seeded and chopped
2 tablespoons paprika
2 tablespoons hoisin sauce
¼ cup lime juice
2 tablespoons light brown sugar
¼ cup mild olive oil
large pinch of sea salt

Gently heat all the ingredients together in a large covered saucepan, stirring, until the sugar has dissolved, then simmer for 12–15 minutes, stirring frequently, until the vegetables are soft.

Ladle the relish into warm, clean, dry jars. Cover with acid-proof lids, seal, and process (see pages 12–13). Store in a cool, dark, dry place for 6 weeks before eating.

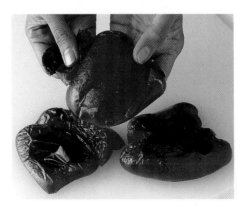

Removing the skins from roasted peppers:
The charred and blistered skins of roasted red bell
peppers should be easy to peel off once cooled.

Roasted Red Peppers in Oil

Roasting adds depth to the flavor of red bell peppers and gives them a delicious smoky taste. Choose peppers that feel heavy for their size, as they will be fleshy. The herbs can easily be adapted according to taste.

MAKES ABOUT 1½ QUARTS

6–8 fleshy red bell peppers, halved lengthwise
2½–3 cups white wine vinegar
2 fresh bay leaves, torn across the middle,
   or some small sprigs of fresh basil
about 1¼ cups olive oil

Broil the red peppers under a hot broiler until the skins are charred and blistered. Leave until cool enough to handle, then discard the cores and seeds and peel off the skins.

Pour the vinegar into a large saucepan and bring to a boil. Place the peppers in the boiling vinegar, cover, return quickly to a boil, and boil for 45–60 seconds. Remove with a slotted spoon and spread out to dry on paper towels.

Pack the peppers into a clean jar, inserting the herbs and covering with oil as you go. Cover completely with oil and rotate the jar to expel all the air. Cover, seal, and process (see pages 12–13). Store in a cool, dark, dry place for 2–3 weeks before eating.

Variation: *Stuffed Red Peppers*
Slice the roasted and blanched peppers into 6 pieces. Place an anchovy fillet on the inside of each piece, then roll up securely. Pack the rolls into the jar, laying a basil leaf and sliver of garlic on each layer and covering with olive oil as you go. Fill the jar, cover, and seal as above.

Serving Suggestion
Serve as an antipasto with cheese, cold meats, and olives; chop and add to salads; or slice and toss with pasta (see page 33).

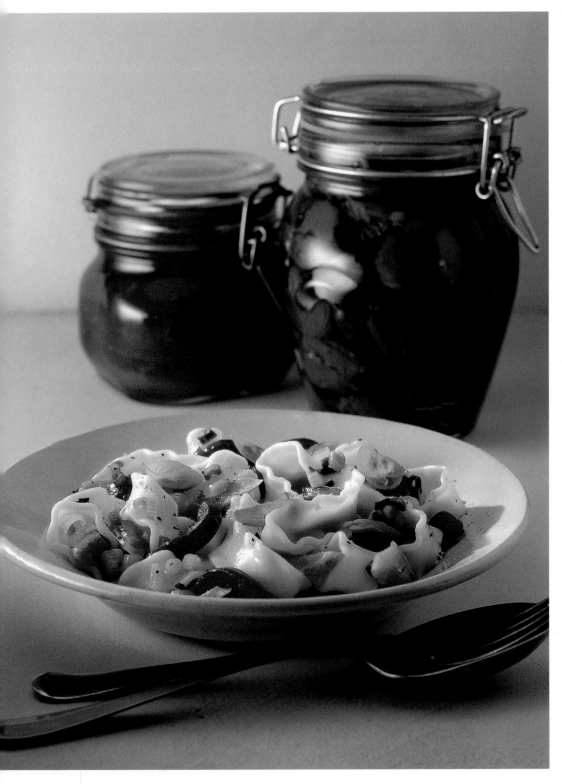

Fettuccine with Smoked Trout, Basil, and Roasted Red Peppers

Some of the best of the Mediterranean preserves can be used as the basis for effortless and delicious dinners. This recipe can be prepared in the time it takes to cook some pasta.

SERVES 4

3 tablespoons oil from Roasted Red Peppers in Oil (see page 32)
3–4 green onions, finely chopped
1 garlic clove, chopped
12 ounces fresh or dried fettuccine
salt
6 Roasted Red Peppers in Oil, halved and sliced
8 ounces smoked trout, flaked
leaves from a small handful of basil, chopped
freshly ground black pepper

Gently heat the oil in a saucepan, add the green onions and garlic, and cook gently until softened but not colored.

Meanwhile, put the fettuccine in a pan of boiling salted water and cook until tender. While the pasta is cooking, add the pepper strips to the onions and garlic and heat for 1 minute, stirring, then add the trout and basil. Continue heating for a another minute, then remove from the heat and season with freshly ground black pepper.

As soon as the pasta is tender, drain, and toss lightly with the red pepper mixture. Serve immediately.

Left: Fettuccine with Smoked Trout, Basil, and Roasted Red Peppers with (at rear) Roasted Red Peppers in Oil and Middle Eastern Stuffed Eggplants in Oil.

Dried Tomatoes in Oil

Oven-dried tomatoes have a delicious, concentrated flavor, and are economical to produce. However, commercial store-bought dried tomatoes in oil can also be used to make Dried Tomato and Cornmeal Rolls (see right) if you are pushed for time.

4½ pounds fleshy, ripe tomatoes
sea salt
bunch of fresh herbs such as basil or thyme and marjoram with a little rosemary (optional)
1 bay leaf or 2–3 sprigs of dried oregano (optional)
4–5 garlic cloves (optional)
virgin olive oil

Preheat the oven to the lowest setting. Line the bottom of the oven with foil to protect it from the drips from the tomatoes.

Halve the tomatoes lengthwise and scoop out the seeds using a teaspoon. As each tomato half is ready, place it, cut side down, on a few thicknesses of paper towels.

Sprinkle salt very lightly on each tomato half, then place them, cut side down, on a wire rack, spacing them slightly apart.

Put the racks in the oven and prop the door very slightly ajar with a skewer (or something similar) so that the tomatoes dry out rather than cook. Leave for 6–12 hours depending on the size of the tomatoes and the temperature of the oven, or until the tomatoes feel dry but are still slightly fleshy (they should not become papery). Remove from the oven and leave to cool.

Loosely pack the tomatoes in clean, dry jars, adding the herbs and garlic if using. Pour in olive oil to cover and rotate the jars to expel any air. Cover, seal, and process the jars (see pages 12–13). Store in a cool, dark, dry place for 2–4 weeks before eating.

Right: Dried Tomatoes in Oil are a visually striking focus for these delicious Cornmeal Rolls.

Dried Tomato and Cornmeal Rolls

MAKES 6–12 ROLLS

3 cups all-purpose flour
1 teaspoon salt
1 cup plus 2 tablespoons cornmeal
1 teaspoon dried oregano
1 teaspoon dry yeast
2 tablespoons oil from Dried Tomatoes in Oil (see left), plus extra for brushing
1 cup plus 2 tablespoons water
¼ cup Dried Tomatoes in Oil, drained and chopped
sea salt

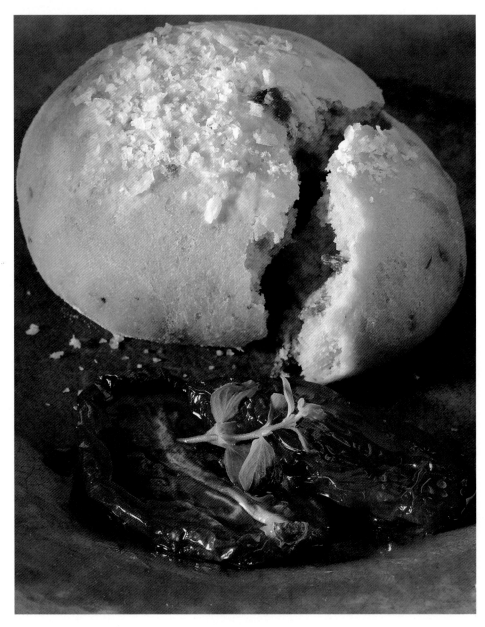

$\mathscr{T}$ OMATOES

Sift 2½ cups flour and the salt into a bowl, then stir in the cornmeal, herbs, and yeast. Make a well in the center and slowly pour in 1 cup plus 2 tablespoons water and the oil, stirring together to make a smooth, sticky dough that is too wet to knead. Cover the bowl and leave in a draft-free place until the dough is doubled in volume and frothy.

Punch down the dough and turn it onto a floured surface. Knead for about 15 minutes, working in as much flour as needed to make a soft dough. Flatten the dough, sprinkle the tomatoes on top, and continue to knead for about 5 minutes, by which time the tomatoes should be evenly distributed.

Lightly flour a baking sheet. Form the dough into 6–12 rolls, place on the baking sheet, and leave the dough to rise in a draft-free place until doubled in volume. Preheat the oven to 425°F.

Brush the rolls with a little extra oil and sprinkle with sea salt. Bake the rolls for 12–20 minutes, depending on size, or until they are risen, lightly browned, and the undersides sound hollow when tapped.

Green Tomato Chutney

Almost everybody who grows tomatoes seems to end up with some green ones. The best way to use these up is to make chutney. The quantity of garlic may seem excessive, but the flavor mellows during cooking and storage.

MAKES ABOUT 2 CUPS

2¼ pounds green tomatoes, coarsely chopped
4 ounces fresh ginger, thinly sliced
3 fresh green chilies, seeded and chopped
23 large garlic cloves, chopped
1 tablespoon brown sugar
1 teaspoon sea salt
2½ cups cider vinegar

Put all the ingredients except the vinegar in a large saucepan, then add half the vinegar

and bring to a boil. Simmer, stirring frequently, for about 20 minutes or until the ingredients are tender. Add the remaining vinegar.

Bring the mixture to a boil again, then simmer until the chutney is well reduced and there is no free liquid.

Ladle into warm, clean, dry jars. Cover with acid-proof lids, seal, and process (see pages 12–13). Store in a cool, dark, dry place for 1 month before eating.

Tomato Ketchup

MAKES ABOUT 5 CUPS

5 pounds ripe tomatoes, chopped
1½ fleshy red bell peppers, cored, seeded, and chopped
2 large red onions, chopped
4 garlic cloves, chopped
1 cup red wine vinegar
1 teaspoon celery or mustard seeds
1 small piece of mace blade
1 teaspoon black peppercorns
¾–1 teaspoon hot paprika
pinch of cayenne pepper
1 teaspoon rock or sea salt
1 tablespoon tarragon vinegar (optional)

Gently cook the tomatoes, peppers, onions and garlic in ½ cup of the red wine vinegar until very soft, then increase the heat and boil vigorously, stirring frequently, until the liquid evaporates and the vegetable mixture becomes very thick.

Use a wooden spoon to press the vegetables against the sides of a nonmetallic sieve. Discard the juice, then return the vegetables to the pan. Tie the celery or mustard seeds, mace, and peppercorns in a square of cheesecloth and add to the pan with the paprika, cayenne, salt, remaining red wine vinegar, and the tarragon vinegar if using. Bring to a boil, then simmer, stirring frequently, until very thick. Remove from the heat and take out the cheesecloth bag.

Pour into warm, clean, dry bottles. Cover with acid-proof lids, seal, and process (see pages 12–13). Process in a boiling water bath for 30 minutes (see pages 12–13). Store in a cool, dark, dry place for 2 weeks before eating and 9–12 months total.

Tomato and Red Pepper Relish

There is relatively little vinegar in this recipe, which makes it a very mild relish. The addition of a little chili makes it more lively. If you are unable to keep the heat sufficiently low, use a heat-diffusing ring.

MAKES ABOUT 3⅔ CUPS

¼ cup olive oil
8 ounces Spanish onion, finely chopped
2 large, fleshy red bell peppers, cored, seeded, and chopped
1 garlic clove, crushed
1 fresh red chili, seeded and finely chopped (optional)
½ teaspoon each ground allspice, ground ginger, paprika, and salt
1 pound ripe tomatoes, peeled and chopped
1¼ cups sugar
⅔ cup white wine vinegar

Heat the oil in a large saucepan, then add the onion and cook gently until very soft. Add the peppers, garlic, chilli if using, spices, and salt and cook for 10 minutes.

Stir in the remaining ingredients, cover, and cook very slowly for at least 1¼ hours or until the relish is thickened but not too thick. Stir occasionally during most of the cooking and more frequently toward the end to prevent the relish from burning.

Ladle into warm, clean, dry jars. Cover with acid-proof lids, seal, and process (see pages 12–13). Store in a cool, dark, dry place for 2 months before eating.

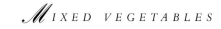

Ratatouille Chutney

This is my chosen proportion of vegetables, but except for the tomatoes, they can be altered according to taste.

MAKES ABOUT 5⅓ CUPS

1¼ tablespoons coriander seeds
2¼ pounds tomatoes, peeled and finely chopped
12 ounces onions, finely chopped
12 ounces eggplants, finely diced
12 ounces zucchini, finely diced
12 ounces red bell peppers, cored, seeded, and finely diced
8 ounces green bell peppers, cored, seeded, and finely diced
3 garlic cloves, crushed
1 tablespoon paprika
1 tablespoon cayenne pepper
1 tablespoon sea salt
1¾ cups sugar
1¼ cups red wine vinegar

Toast the coriander seeds in a heavy-based, preferably nonstick skillet for ½–1 minute over low heat, stirring to prevent them from burning, until they are fragrant. Remove the seeds from the pan and crush them lightly with the end of a rolling pin. Set aside.

Gently heat the vegetables, garlic, paprika, cayenne, crushed coriander, and salt together in a covered saucepan for about 10 minutes, stirring occasionally, until the juices run. Uncover and bring to a boil, then simmer for 1 hour or until the vegetables are soft and most of the liquid has evaporated.

Over low heat, stir in the sugar and vinegar until the sugar has dissolved, then simmer for another hour, stirring occasionally, until the chutney is very thick and there is no free liquid.

Ladle the chutney into warm, clean, dry jars. Cover the jars with acid-proof lids, seal, and process (see pages 12–13). Store the chutney in a cool, dark, dry place for at least 1 month before eating.

Italian Garden Pickle

As the name suggests, this colorful pickle uses all the vegetables that would be found in an Italian country garden.

MAKES ABOUT 7½ CUPS

8 ounces red onions
1 red bell pepper, cored, seeded, and cut into chunks
1 eggplant, cut into thick matchsticks
8 ounces small zucchini, cut into thick matchsticks
1 small fennel bulb, cut into wedges
4 ounces button mushrooms
¾ cup sea salt
4 ounces cherry tomatoes
4–6 garlic cloves, sliced
7 tablespoons walnut oil
3 cups white wine vinegar
2–3 small fresh bay leaves or sprigs of rosemary
several sprigs of fresh tarragon
2 teaspoons black peppercorns, lightly crushed

Trim the red onions, leaving the root end intact, then cut lengthwise into thick wedges. Layer all the vegetables, except the tomatoes and the garlic, in a nonmetallic bowl, sprinkling salt between the layers. Pour in 7½ cups water, use a plate to keep the vegetables submerged, and leave in a cool place overnight.

Drain the vegetables and rinse them well, then spread them out on paper towels and leave to dry thoroughly.

Transfer the vegetables to a bowl and stir in the tomatoes, garlic, and walnut oil. Pour a thin layer of vinegar into the bottom of a large, clean, dry jar and add a bay leaf or rosemary sprig and a tarragon sprig.

Using a spoon, pack the vegetables into the jar, adding peppercorns and the remaining herbs as you go so that they are evenly distributed. Pour vinegar over each layer. Cover the vegetables completely with vinegar, rotate the jar to expel any air, then cover with an acid-proof lid, seal, and

process (see pages 12–13). Store in a cool, dark, dry place for 1 month before eating.

Serving Suggestion
Serve lightly dressed with oil as part of an antipasto or with cold meats.

Indonesian Cauliflower Pickle

This is a nutty, spicy vegetable pickle.

MAKES ABOUT 2 CUPS

2 plump garlic cloves, crushed
1-ounce piece of fresh ginger, peeled and grated
2 teaspoons ground turmeric
3 tablespoons peanut oil
⅔ cup Spiced Vinegar (see page 139)
6 ounces cauliflower florets
1 large red bell pepper, cored, seeded, and chopped
½ cucumber, sliced
1–2 fresh green chilies, seeded
¼ cup sesame seeds
10 tablespoons dark or light brown sugar
1 cup salted peanuts, chopped

In a large saucepan, gently heat the garlic, ginger, and turmeric in the oil for about 5 minutes, stirring occasionally, until fragrant. Stir in the vinegar.

Bring to a boil, then add the cauliflower, bell pepper, and cucumber and return to a boil. Cover and simmer until the vegetables are tender. Stir in the remaining ingredients.

Ladle the chutney into warm, clean, dry jars. Rotate the jars to expel any air. Cover with acid-proof lids, seal, and process (see pages 12–13). Store in a cool, dark, dry place for 2 months before eating.

Serving Suggestion
This pickle goes well with hard cheeses.

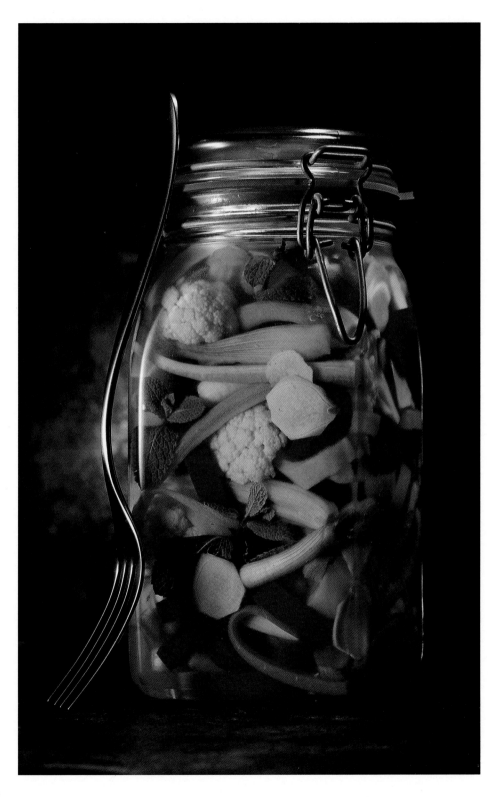

Pickled Vegetables with Ginger and Mint

Ginger, mint, and rice vinegar produce deliciously delicate pickled vegetables. Rice vinegar is available from specialty food shops and some supermarkets. It is mild, so it does not have the same preserving properties as other vinegars. You should therefore use the pickle within 6 months.

MAKES 5 CUPS

2¼ pounds mixed vegetables, such as small fennel bulbs, small carrots, celery sticks, red and yellow bell peppers, plump green onions, and cauliflower
1 cup sea salt
several sprigs of fresh mint
¼-ounce piece of plump fresh ginger, peeled and thinly sliced
3½ cups rice vinegar

Prepare the vegetables: Cut the fennel into slim wedges; quarter the carrots and celery sticks; core, seed, and slice the peppers; remove most of the green part from the green onions; divide the cauliflower into small florets.

Layer the vegetables with the salt in a large nonmetallic bowl. Cover with a lightly weighted plate to press the vegetables slightly and leave for 8–12 hours.

Rinse the vegetables under cold running water, drain well, and dry thoroughly on paper towels. Pack into clean, dry jars, adding mint and ginger at regular intervals.

Pour in vinegar to cover the vegetables and rotate the jars to expel any air, then cover with acid-proof lids, seal, and process (see pages 12–13). Store in a cool, dark, dry place for 1 month before using.

Left: Pickled Vegetables with Ginger and Mint is made using rice vinegar for a preserve that is deliciously delicate.

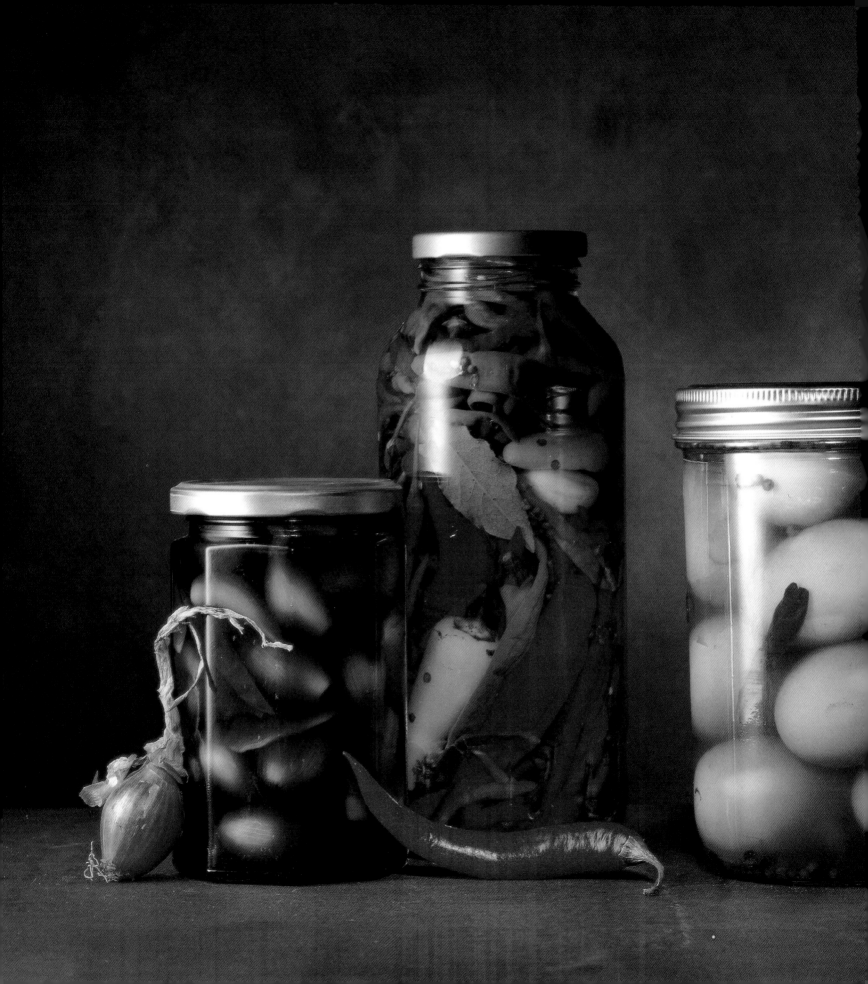

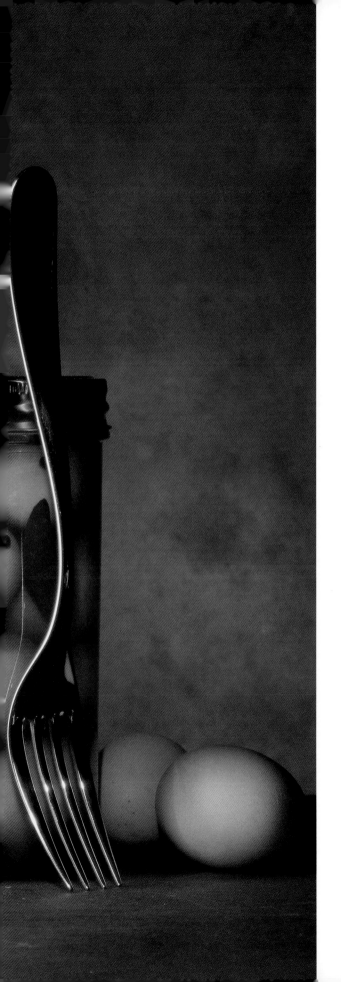

$\mathscr{H}$OT, $\mathscr{S}$PICY, AND $\mathscr{S}$ALTY

Preserves made from hot, spicy, or salty ingredients come from all around the world. The preserves in this chapter will really add a lift and give a flavor boost to the dishes you serve them with. They range from a fiery Red Curry Paste (see page 40) from Thailand to Japanese Pickled Ginger (see page 48) and Harissa (see page 42), a great staple of Tunisian cooking. You can increase or decrease the quantity of chilies you use in each recipe depending on whether you like fiery food or just a hint of heat. Because they are generally used in small quantities, the preserves on the following pages will last quite a while.

Left, from left to right: Chinese-Style Shallots, Pickled Mixed Chilies, and Eggs in Spiced Vinegar.

Piquant Sauce

This tangy sauce can be used as a condiment to liven up many savory dishes.

MAKES ABOUT 2½ CUPS

**1 head of garlic, divided into cloves
   and chopped
1 shallot, chopped
6 anchovy fillets, drained and chopped
2½ cups red wine vinegar
1 tablespoon cayenne pepper**

Stir all the ingredients together in a nonmetallic bowl. Cover and leave in a cool place for 2 weeks, stirring 2 or 3 times a day to disperse the flavors.

Strain through a nonmetallic sieve lined with a double thickness of cheesecloth, then

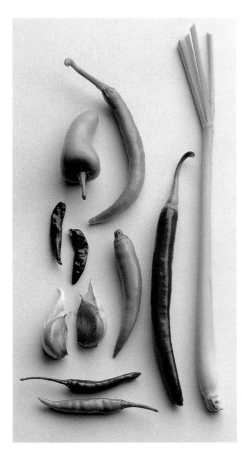

pour into bottles. Cover with acid-proof lids, seal, and process (see pages 12–13). Store the sauce in a cool, dark, dry place for at least 1 month before using.

Serving Suggestion
Enhances the flavor of plain fish, fish soups, or casseroles; use in white sauces.

Mediterranean Spread

Use French whole-grain mustard, as it is usually more piquant than other types.

MAKES ABOUT ⅔ CUP

**2-ounce can anchovy fillets in oil
1 cup Dried Tomatoes in Oil (see page 34),
   drained
1 cup capers
2½ tablespoons pitted oil-cured black olives,
   drained
2 garlic cloves, whole
1 teaspoon French whole-grain mustard
pinch of ground allspice
1 teaspoon brandy
about 5 tablespoons olive oil, plus extra
   for covering
freshly ground black pepper**

Put the anchovy fillets and their oil, the dried tomatoes, capers, olives, garlic, mustard, and allspice in a food processor or blender and process to make a fairly smooth paste. Briefly mix in the brandy, then, with the motor running, slowly pour in the olive oil. Add pepper to taste.

Spoon the spread into a clean, dry jar, pour a little olive oil on top, and cover tightly. Store in a cool, dark, dry place for at least 2 days before using. This will keep in the refrigerator, covered, for 6–8 weeks.

Left, clockwise from top left: Jalapeño, cayenne pepper, lemongrass, Tabasco chili, orange chili, red and green chilies, garlic, and serrano chilies.

Serving Suggestion
Spread on fresh crusty bread, then top with a cool soft cheese such as goat's cheese; use a little to top broiled beef, lamb, or pork steaks and chops or grilled eggplant slices; insert under the skin of chicken before roasting; mash with the yolks of hard-boiled eggs and spoon back into the whites for delicious stuffed eggs.

Red Curry Paste

This is a typical Thai red curry paste; look for shrimp paste in your local Asian or specialty food market.

MAKES ABOUT ¼ CUP

**1 teaspoon cumin seeds
1 tablespoon coriander seeds
1 teaspoon black peppercorns
4 garlic cloves, chopped
1-inch piece of fresh ginger, peeled and
   finely chopped
1 teaspoon finely grated lime zest
2 stalks lemongrass, bulbs only, finely chopped
about 8 dried red chilies, seeded if desired (to
   reduce the heat), chopped
2 teaspoons shrimp paste**

Heat a heavy-based, preferably nonstick, skillet over low heat, then add the cumin and coriander seeds and heat for ½–1 minute or until fragrant. Transfer to a mortar or small blender and crush lightly. Add the remaining ingredients and pound or mix into a paste.

Spoon the mixture into a clean, dry jar. Cover and store in a cool, dark, dry place for at least 2 days before using, then keep in the refrigerator for 6–8 weeks.

Serving Suggestion
Use to add zest to casseroles and sauces; spread sparingly on meats before broiling or on bread for savory sandwiches.

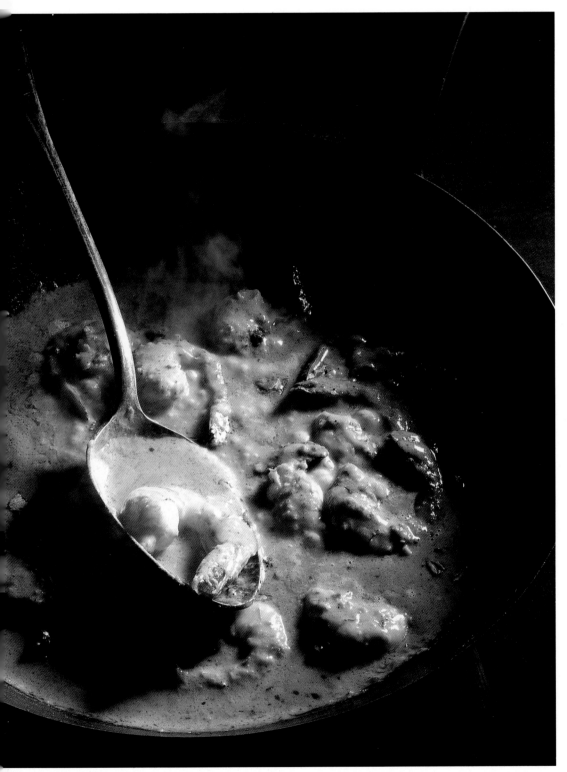

Thai Shrimp Curry

Unlike Indian curries, which need long, slow simmering, Thai curries need very little cooking time. The fish sauce and coconut milk can be found in most good supermarkets and specialty or ethnic food shops.

SERVES 2-3
2 tablespoons peanut oil
1 plump garlic clove, finely chopped
1 tablespoon Red Curry Paste (see page 40)
1 cup coconut milk
2 tablespoons fish sauce
1 teaspoon sugar (optional)
12 raw large shrimp, about 3 inches long,
shells removed but tails left intact
zest of 2–3 limes, finely grated
10 basil leaves, torn

Heat the oil in a skillet over medium heat, then add the garlic and cook until pale gold and fragrant. Stir in the curry paste and heat briefly, then stir in half the coconut milk, the fish sauce, and the sugar if using.

Add the shrimp and cook, turning once, for 2–3 minutes or until they begin to turn opaque. Add the remaining coconut milk and the lime zest and continue cooking until the shrimp are cooked through. Add the torn basil leaves and serve with boiled regular or basmati rice.

Left: The flavors of plump shrimp, coconut milk, fresh basil, and Red Curry Paste mingle in this fragrant Thai Shrimp Curry.

41

Harissa

Harissa, or "arhissa," as this is sometimes called, is a fiery paste made from chilies. It is primarily associated with Tunisian cooking, but it is also used in Algerian and Moroccan cuisines. It is often served as a condiment in a small dish with a small spoon. It is also used in cooking and as an accompaniment to couscous.

MAKES ABOUT ¼ CUP

1 ounce dried red chilies
1 garlic clove, chopped
1 teaspoon coriander seeds
1 teaspoon cumin seeds
1 teaspoon caraway seeds
pinch of sea salt
3 tablespoons olive oil

Put the chilies in a bowl, cover with hot water, and leave to soak for 1 hour.

Drain the chilies and put them in a mortar, spice grinder, or small blender with the garlic, the coriander, cumin, and caraway seeds, and the salt. Mix into a paste, then stir in 2 tablespoons olive oil.

Transfer to a small jar and pour a little oil over the surface. Cover and store in a cool, dark, dry place for 1 day before using. This lasts for about 4 months.

Serving Suggestion
Harissa is a versatile seasoning that will add life to many savory dishes; add it to meat, poultry, or vegetable casseroles, saffron-flavored fish soups and stews, stewed red bell peppers and tomatoes used as a base for poached eggs, or add to salad dressings.

Mix a little harissa with peeled, seeded, and finely chopped well-flavored tomatoes, add a pinch of salt, and serve as a dipping sauce for kebabs.

Right: Fresh "Hot" Tomato and Red Pepper Relish is quickly made from homemade pantry preserves and brings any dish to life.

Fresh "Hot" Tomato and Red Pepper Relish

When you want to add a little heat to dishes, simply dip a small spoon into a pot of harissa instead of seeding and chopping chilies. For this vibrant relish, you can make use of another recipe in this book, Roasted Red Peppers in Oil (page 32). If you do not have any on hand, roast a fresh red bell pepper until charred and blistered, then peel it (see page 32). When you drain off the oil, save it for making salad dressings.

SERVES 4

18 ounces well-flavored tomatoes
1–2 garlic cloves, unpeeled
2 halves Roasted Red Peppers in Oil
    (see page 32), chopped
1–2 teaspoons Harissa (see left)
sea salt
2 tablespoons oil from the Roasted Red
    Peppers or 2 tablespoons virgin olive oil

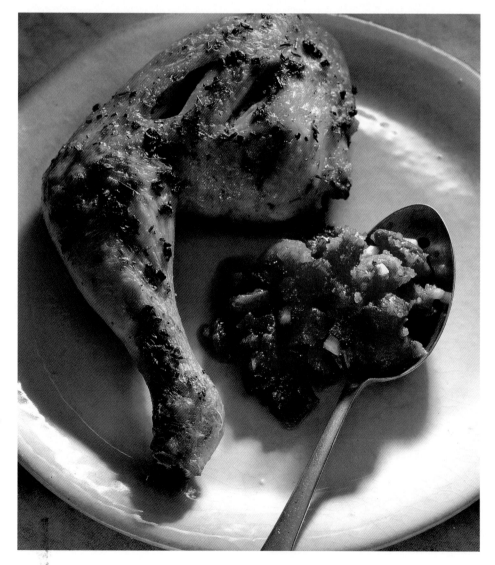

Preheat the broiler to medium-high.

Broil the tomatoes and garlic cloves, turning them occasionally, until charred and blistered; the garlic should be soft. Leave until cool enough to handle, then peel, seed, and coarsely chop the tomatoes; peel and chop the garlic.

Mix together the tomatoes, garlic, peppers, harissa, salt to taste, and oil. Set aside for 2 hours.

Drain off the oil and spoon into a clean, dry jar. Cover, seal, and process, then store in a cool, dark, dry place for at least 1 month before use.

Serving Suggestion
Serve with broiled meats or poultry; baked, poached, grilled, or fried fish; on bread.

Tomatillo and Chili Relish

Tomatillos are sometimes called Mexican green tomatoes, but they are not related to tomatoes. In fact, tomatillos are a relative of the Cape gooseberry. Although green and acidic when unripe (like most fruits), when ripe and bright yellow, they have a papery outer covering similar to the Cape gooseberry. The flavor is slightly reminiscent of apple and it develops on cooking. Modify the heat of this relish by adjusting the number of chilies and removing the chili seeds for a milder flavor.

MAKES ABOUT ⅔ CUP

8 fresh tomatillos, loose skins removed
10 fresh green chilies
3 garlic cloves
1 onion, quartered
6 tablespoons sugar
5 tablespoons cider vinegar
1 teaspoon ground cinnamon
1 teaspoon sea salt

Mix all the ingredients in a blender or food processor to the texture you require. Pour into a small saucepan and simmer, stirring frequently, for about 20 minutes or until the relish is thick.

Pour into a warm, clean, dry jar, loosely cover with an acid-proof lid, and process in a water bath for 20 minutes (see page 13). Store in a cool, dark, dry place for 1 month before using. Once opened, refrigerate. If not processed in a water bath, it will keep for 1 month total in the refrigerator.

Serving Suggestion
Eat with Mexican-style dishes, or poultry.

Pickled Mixed Chilies

A mixture of colors and sizes gives added interest to the look and flavor of this recipe, but it is still worth making if you can only find chilies that are all the same.

MAKES ABOUT 1 QUART

8 ounces mixed fresh chilies, whole
1 small dried red chili, crushed
3 garlic cloves
1 teaspoon coriander seeds, lightly crushed
1 teaspoon whole cloves
2 bay leaves
2½ cups white wine vinegar, warmed
2 teaspoons superfine sugar

Place the whole fresh chilies in a small saucepan, cover with water, and bring to a simmer. Continue simmering for 5 minutes.

Using a slotted spoon, transfer the chilies to paper towels to dry, then pack them into a clean, dry jar. Add the remaining ingredients and rotate the jar to dissolve the sugar and to expel any air. Cover with an acid-proof lid, seal, and process (see pages 12–13). Store the pickled chilies in a cool, dark, dry place for 2 weeks, shaking the jar occasionally, before eating.

Hot Pepper Sauce

The exact degree of heat in this colorful curry-flavored sauce will be determined by the type of chilies you use (small ones are generally hotter than large ones), whether the seeds are left in or removed, and, of course, the number used. The amount of mustard powder used influences the flavor of the sauce as well.

MAKES 3½ CUPS

1 small green mango
2 onions, finely chopped
2 garlic cloves, finely chopped
10–12 fresh red chilies, seeded if desired and chopped
1 teaspoon curry powder
½ teaspoon ground turmeric
2 teaspoons table salt
2 cups white wine vinegar
¼ cup dry English mustard

Put the whole mango in a large saucepan and just cover with water, then bring to a boil. Cover and simmer for about 10 minutes. Drain and leave the mango until cool enough to handle, then peel and coarsely chop.

Put the mango, onions, garlic, chilies, curry powder, turmeric, salt, and 1¾ cups of the vinegar in a saucepan and simmer gently for 15 minutes, stirring occasionally.

In a small bowl, stir the remaining vinegar into the mustard, then stir the mixture into the pan and bring to a boil. Remove from the heat. Pour into a warm, clean, dry jar. Cover with an acid-proof lid, seal, and process (see pages 12–13). Store in a cool, dark, dry place for 1 month before eating.

Serving Suggestion
Use in casseroles, marinades, and salad dressings and as a relish.

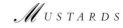

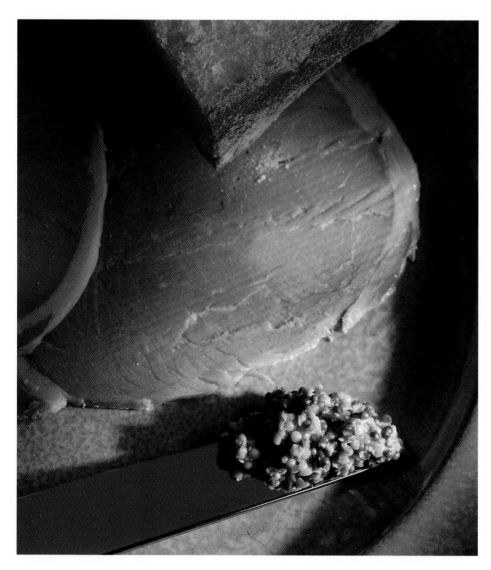

Tarragon Mustard

Unlike mustard made from English mustard powder, which is ready to eat after being left to stand for a short while, this mustard should be kept for at least 2 weeks to allow the flavors to mature.

MAKES ABOUT ¾ CUP

⅓ cup plus 2 teaspoons yellow mustard seeds
scant 1 cup black mustard seeds
7 tablespoons dry white wine
1 tablespoon white wine vinegar
leaves from a small bunch of fresh tarragon,
 finely chopped
1 tablespoon sea salt

Grind the mustard seeds in a spice grinder or small blender as finely as you like – the finer the grind, the hotter the mustard. Transfer them to a nonmetallic bowl, then stir in 3 tablespoons water and leave for 10 minutes before adding the remaining ingredients. Stir together well.

Transfer the mustard to clean, dry jars. Cover loosely with acid-proof lids and leave to stand overnight at room temperature. The next day, stir, then cover tightly and store in a cool, dark, dry place for at least 2 weeks before eating.

Mustard Dipping Sauce

This sauce is thinner than the Sweet Mustard Sauce that follows this recipe.

MAKES ABOUT ¾ CUP

6 tablespoons soy sauce
3 tablespoons Dijon mustard
6 tablespoons sake
several drops of Tabasco sauce

In a small bowl, whisk the soy sauce into the mustard, then whisk in the sake. Add Tabasco sauce to taste and whisk together.

Grainy Mustard

The mustard seeds needed for this recipe can be found in Indian, Chinese, and health food stores.

MAKES ABOUT 1 CUP

generous ½ cup black mustard seeds
⅓ cup plus 2 teaspoons yellow mustard seeds
½ cup white wine vinegar
1 shallot, finely chopped
1 tablespoon sea salt

Above: Grainy Mustard is particularly delicious eaten with cold ham and fresh bread.

Soak the mustard seeds in the vinegar in a nonmetallic bowl for 24 hours.

Stir in the shallot and salt and crush the seeds into a coarse paste using the end of a rolling pin, adding a little more vinegar if necessary. Transfer to clean, dry jars, cover tightly with acid-proof lids, and seal. Store in a cool, dark, dry place for at least 2 weeks before using.

Pour, into a clean, dry bottle, then cover, seal, and process. The sauce can be used immediately but is best left for up to 4 hours. Shake well before using. Store in a cool, dark, dry place for up to 1 year.

Sweet Mustard Sauce

Mirin, Japanese sweetened sake, adds a touch of sweetness to this versatile sauce. You can buy mirin from good supermarkets or specialty food stores.

MAKES ABOUT 1 CUP

3 tablespoons rice wine vinegar
6 tablespoons Dijon mustard
6 tablespoons mild oil, such as mild olive
    or sunflower oil
3 tablespoons mirin

In a small bowl, whisk the vinegar into the mustard, then slowly pour in the oil, still whisking (see below). Add the mirin and whisk together.

  Pour into a clean, dry bottle, cover, seal, and process (see pages 12–13). Leave for 2–4 hours and shake before using. This will keep in a cool, dark, dry place for 6 months.

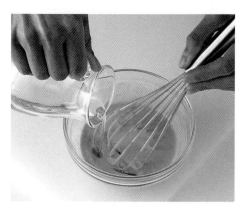

Adding the oil: Pour the oil into the vinegar and mustard mixture in a slow, steady stream, whisking constantly.

Eggs in Spiced Vinegar

Eggs in Spiced Vinegar are easy to prepare and versatile. As the eggs are used, they can be replaced with freshly cooked ones, but try to ease these to the bottom of the jar so that the older eggs are eaten first.

MAKES 5⅓ CUPS

3½ cups cider vinegar or
    white wine vinegar
1-inch piece of fresh ginger
1 tablespoon coriander seeds
2 dried red chilies
2 garlic cloves, crushed (optional)
1½ tablespoons black peppercorns
12 hard-cooked eggs, peeled

Put all the ingredients except the eggs in a large saucepan and bring to a boil, then simmer for about 10 minutes. Remove from the heat, cover, and leave to cool.

  Pack the eggs into clean, dry jars, then strain in the vinegar through a nonmetallic sieve to cover the eggs completely. Cover with acid-proof lids, seal, and process (see pages 12–13). Store the eggs in a cool, dark, dry place for 6–8 weeks before eating or up to 1 year.

Chinese-Style Shallots

These shallots provide an interesting alternative to pickled onions. Small onions and garlic can be preserved too.

MAKES 4 CUPS

3 pounds shallots
1 dried red chili
3 slices fresh ginger
about 2½ cups soy sauce,
    preferably shoyu

Place the shallots in a heatproof bowl, pour boiling water over, and leave for 2 minutes.

Drain the shallots, then trim and peel them. Pack into a clean, dry 1-quart jar with the chili and ginger. Pour in soy sauce to cover completely. Cover, seal, and process the jar (see pages 12–13). Store the shallots in a cool, dark, dry place for 4–6 months before eating.

Indian Pickled Onions

The red wine vinegar in this recipe turns the onions pink. To make peeling the onions easy, cut off the tip ends, pour boiling water over them, and leave them for a minute or so, then drain and rinse quickly under running cold water. Use a stainless steel knife to prevent discoloration.

MAKES ABOUT 5 CUPS

1 pound pickling onions
½ cup sea salt
2 cups red wine vinegar
2 garlic cloves, sliced
2 dried red chilies

Cut a deep cross from the top to the bottom of each onion, but leave them attached at the root ends. Dissolve the salt in 2½ cups water in a nonmetallic bowl, then add the onions, cover, and leave for one day at room temperature, stirring occasionally.

  Drain and rinse the onions thoroughly, then dry well on paper towels. Pack the onions into a 1-liter jar. If there are too many onions, they may be reserved and used in cooking.

  Mix together the vinegar, garlic, and chilies and pour over the onions to cover them completely; if the onions float, put crumpled waxed paper in the jar to keep them submerged. Rotate the jar to expel any air, then cover with acid-proof lids, seal, and process (see pages 12–13). Store the onions in a cool, dark, dry place for 1 month before eating.

Indian Carrot Sticks in Oil

Mustard oil is used a great deal in Bengali and Kashmiri cooking. It has a split personality, smelling fiery when cold, but losing its pungency when heated and becoming slightly sweet.

MAKES 1 QUART

1 pound carrots, cut into matchsticks
at least 1 tablespoon black mustard seeds,
** or extra, to taste**
1 teaspoon cayenne pepper
1 teaspoon ground turmeric
2 cups mustard oil or peanut oil,
** to cover, warmed if liked**

Bring a large saucepan of salted water to a boil, add the carrots, and continue boiling for about 5 minutes. Drain well, then spread out on paper towels to dry.

In a small bowl, crush the mustard seeds with the end of a rolling pin, so that they split in half or into quarters. Place in a small bowl and mix together with the cayenne pepper, turmeric, and about ½ cup oil.

Using a spoon, pack the carrots into a clean, dry jar. Pour in the flavored oil and top up with more oil to cover the carrots completely. Rotate the jar to expel all the air bubbles. Cover, seal, and process (see pages 12–13). Store in a cool, dark, dry place for 1 month, shaking the jar daily for the first 10 days or so, before eating. Shake the jar before serving the carrots.

Serving Suggestion
Serve with cocktails, with Indian food, or as an accompaniment to cold roast meats, pâtés, and hard cheeses.

Right: Serve Indian Carrot Sticks with Indian-style dinners or use to perk up Western foods.

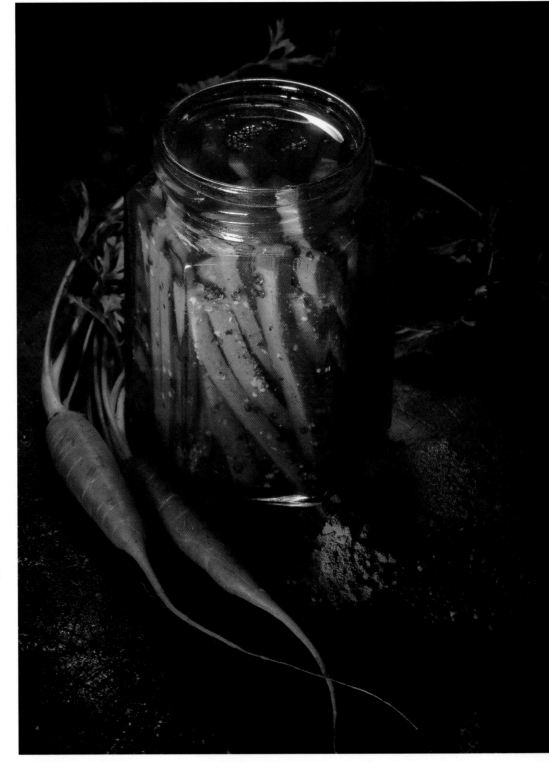

MIXED VEGETABLES

Creole Chow-Chow

Chinese migrant railroad workers introduced this hot pickled chow to American cuisine in the mid-nineteenth-century. It is not unlike Indian-spiced piccalilli.

MAKES ABOUT 4 QUARTS

8 ounces white cabbage, shredded
1 pound whole French beans
2 red bell peppers, cored, seeded, and diced
1 green bell pepper, cored, seeded, and diced
1 pound cucumber, chopped
1 small cauliflower, broken into florets
1½ pounds green tomatoes, chopped
8 ounces pearl or pickling onions
5 tablespoons sea salt
2½ quarts cider vinegar
2 ounces fresh horseradish, grated
8 garlic cloves, crushed
2 tablespoons black mustard seeds
⅓ cup Dijon mustard
2 tablespoons plus 1 teaspoon turmeric
¾ cup plus 2 tablespoons light brown sugar
⅔ cup olive oil or sunflower oil

Layer the vegetables and salt in a large nonmetallic colander and leave to drain for about 12 hours, stirring occasionally.

Place the rest of the ingredients in a large saucepan, stir together, and bring to a boil. Simmer for 5 minutes, stirring constantly. Add the vegetables, without rinsing, and return to a boil. Simmer for 15–20 minutes ensuring that the vegetables remain crisp. Pack into clean, dry jars, cover, seal, and process (see pages 12–13). Store in a cool, dark, dry place for 2 weeks before eating.

Serving Suggestion
Serve with cold roast meats, mature cheeses, and fresh, crusty bread.

Mixed Vegetable Pickle

Don't feel you have to use the selection of vegetables I have given; omit some or use substitutes according to your taste.

You can use a crinkle-edged cutter to slice the vegetables and layer them by variety, or by color, in the jar to make an extremely attractive, as well as delicious, pickle.

MAKES ½ CUP

4 fresh or dried red chilies
2 blades of mace
1½ cinnamon sticks
8 allspice berries
2 bay leaves, torn
about 5 cups white wine vinegar
sea salt
about 9 ounces carrots, cut into ½-inch slices
4 ounces baby corn
1 celery root bulb, or 8 ounces small turnips, cut into ½-inch slices
4 celery stalks, cut into ½-inch slices
1 large red bell pepper, cored, seeded, quartered, and cut into ½-inch slices
9 ounces broccoli florets
3½ ounces snowpeas or French beans, topped and tailed
5 ounces pickling onions

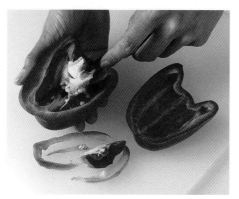

Preparing red peppers: Cut out and discard the core along with any seeds, before removing the white veins.

Place the chilies, mace, cinnamon, allspice berries, and bay leaves in a saucepan, pour in the vinegar, bring to the boiling point, then boil for 2 minutes. Remove from the heat, cover, and leave overnight.

Add the carrots, corn, celery root or turnips, and celery to a large saucepan of boiling salted water and boil for 10 minutes. Add the remaining vegetables and boil for 7–10 minutes or until they are just tender.

Drain the vegetables and spread out to dry on paper towels. Strain the vinegar, then pour a little into a clean, dry jar. Spoon the vegetables into the jar, adding a little vinegar. Cover the vegetables with vinegar and rotate the jar to expel any air. Cover with an acid-proof lid, seal, and process (see pages 12–13). Store in a cool, dark, dry place for 1–3 months before eating.

Easy Pickle

This easy-to-make pickle is ready for eating after 24 hours and keeps for up to 1 year.

MAKES 2⅔ CUPS

1½ cups onions or 1 small Spanish onion, thinly sliced
4 celery stalks, thinly sliced
2 small cooking apples, peeled, cored, and thinly sliced
½ cup soy sauce
½ cup medium-dry sherry
1 teaspoon chili powder
1 cup white wine vinegar

Pack the onions, celery, and apples into a clean, dry jar. In a small bowl, stir together the soy sauce, sherry, and chili powder, then pour over the vegetables. Cover with vinegar and rotate the jar to expel any air bubbles.

Cover the jar with an acid-proof lid, seal, and process (see pages 12–13), then shake it to mix in the vinegar. Store in a cool, dark, dry place for 24 hours before eating.

Pickled Garlic in Oil

This mellows over time. After 3 or 4 months it tastes like lightly poached garlic and is good with cold meats and cheeses. After 6 months it can easily be crushed to add to vegetable and meat dishes or to meat cooking juices to make a quick sauce. Nigella and garam masala are available from Indian markets and some supermarkets.

MAKES ABOUT ⅔ CUP

8 ounces garlic cloves
3 tablespoons fennel seeds
1 tablespoon black peppercorns
1 tablespoon garam masala
1 tablespoon black onion seeds (nigella)
1 teaspoon chili powder
1 tablespoon sea salt
about ¾ cup peanut oil

Pack the garlic cloves into a jar and add the spices and salt. Pour in enough oil to cover the garlic completely, then cover, seal, and process (see pages 12–13).

Leave in a sunny or warm place for 1 week, rotating the jar several times a day, then leave for another week. Transfer to room temperature and store in a cool, dark, dry place for at least 2 months before eating.

Japanese Pickled Ginger

Japanese pickled ginger comes in two forms: *gari*, also known as *amuzu-shoga*, which is yellowish or delicate salmon pink, depending on the length of preservation, and *beni-shoga*, which is dyed garish pink.

MAKES 1 CUP

8-ounce piece of fresh ginger, peeled and cut
    into wafer-thin slices with a sharp knife or a
    mandoline
sea salt

1 tablespoon sugar
1 cup rice vinegar
few drops of red food coloring (optional)

Place the ginger in a small bowl of very cold water to soak for 30 minutes.

Drain the ginger, then add it to a saucepan of boiling water. Return to a boil, then drain and leave the ginger to cool.

Put the ginger slices into a clean, dry jar, sprinkling them with a little salt.

In a saucepan, gently heat the sugar in the vinegar, stirring, until it has dissolved. Add the red coloring, if using, and pour over the ginger to cover completely; rotate the jar to expel any air bubbles. Cover with an acid-proof lid, seal, and process (see pages 12–13). Store in a cool, dark, dry place or in the refrigerator at least 2 weeks before eating. This will keep for up to 3 months.

Serving Suggestion
Traditionally served in a tiny pile with sushi and sashimi, pickled ginger also goes well with other seafood dishes and poultry.

Ginger Wine

MAKES 2 CUPS

6-inch piece of fresh ginger, peeled and chopped
2 cups rice wine

Put the ginger in a clean, dry bottle or jar. Pour in the rice wine, cover, and leave in a warm place for at least 2 weeks, shaking the jar occasionally, before drinking. Strain the wine when it has reached the flavor intensity you like, or top up with more wine once some has been drunk. This wine will keep indefinitely.

Serving Suggestion
Drink on its own or add to salad dressings, stir-fries or fruit salads.

Ginger and Peach Chutney

This is a lively fruit chutney with just a hint of spice. The combination of peaches, ginger, and spices makes for a tangy and refreshing blend of flavors.

MAKES ABOUT 4⅔ CUPS

2¼ pounds peaches, peeled, quartered,
    and pitted
2½ cups white wine vinegar
1¼ cups light brown sugar
⅔ cup preserved ginger in syrup, chopped
⅔ cup pitted dried dates, chopped
⅔ cup plump raisins
1¼ cups sliced almonds
2 onions, finely chopped
3 plump garlic cloves, chopped
grated zest and juice of 2 oranges
1 teaspoon ground allspice
1 teaspoon ground cinnamon
2 teaspoons sea salt

Put all the ingredients in a large saucepan and heat gently, stirring, until the sugar has dissolved. Bring to a boil, then cover and simmer for about 1½ hours, stirring frequently, until there is no free liquid and the chutney is quite thick.

Carefully ladle the chutney into warm, clean, dry jars, then cover with acid-proof lids, seal, and process (see pages 12–13). Store in a cool, dark, dry place for at least 2 months before eating.

Serving Suggestion
This chutney is excellent with ripe Camembert and hard cheeses and makes a good accompaniment to smoked chicken or hot or cold roast chicken, as well as lamb, pork, ham, and game.

Spiced Pineapple Chutney

Using only fresh fruit produces a really fruity-tasting chutney with a lightly spicy flavor.

MAKES ABOUT 2 CUPS

4–5 cardamom seeds
2 pineapples, about 2 pounds
 10 ounces total
½ cup white wine vinegar
1 teaspoon ground cinnamon
2 teaspoons curry powder
½ teaspoon ground ginger
½ teaspoon ground cloves
¾ cup plus 2 tablespoons sugar

Toast the cardamom seeds in a heavy-based, preferably nonstick skillet for ½–1 minute over low heat, stirring to prevent them from burning, until fragrant. Remove the seeds and crush them with the end of a rolling pin. Set aside.

Peel the pineapples, taking care to remove all the eyes. Slice the pineapple, cut out the core, and chop the flesh quite finely, collecting any juices that are released during the preparation.

Put any juices, the vinegar, cardamom, and remaining spices in a large saucepan, bring to a boil, and simmer gently for 5 minutes. Add the pineapple and simmer for about 20 minutes or until tender.

Over low heat, stir in the sugar until it has dissolved, then raise the heat and boil, stirring occasionally, until the chutney is thick and there is no free liquid.

Ladle into warm, clean, dry jars. Cover with acid-proof lids, seal, and process (see pages 12–13). Store in a cool, dark, dry place for 1 month before eating.

Right: Spiced Pineapple Chutney goes well with hot and cold ham, pork, turkey, chicken, and cheese.

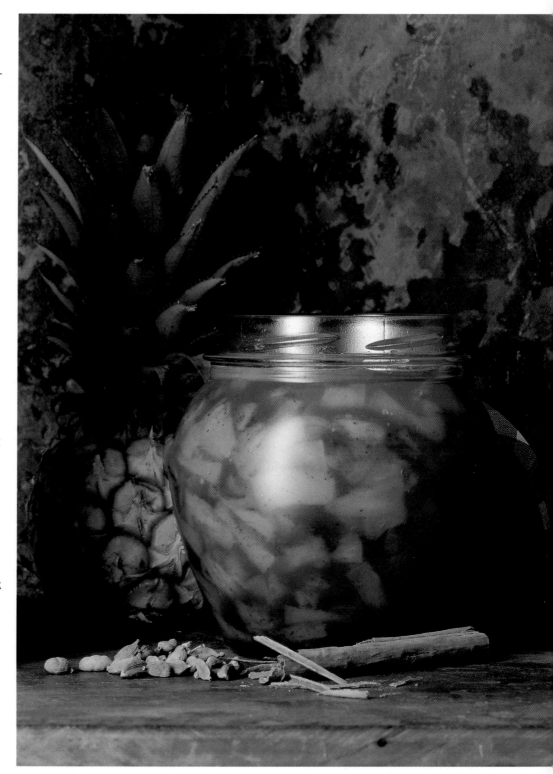

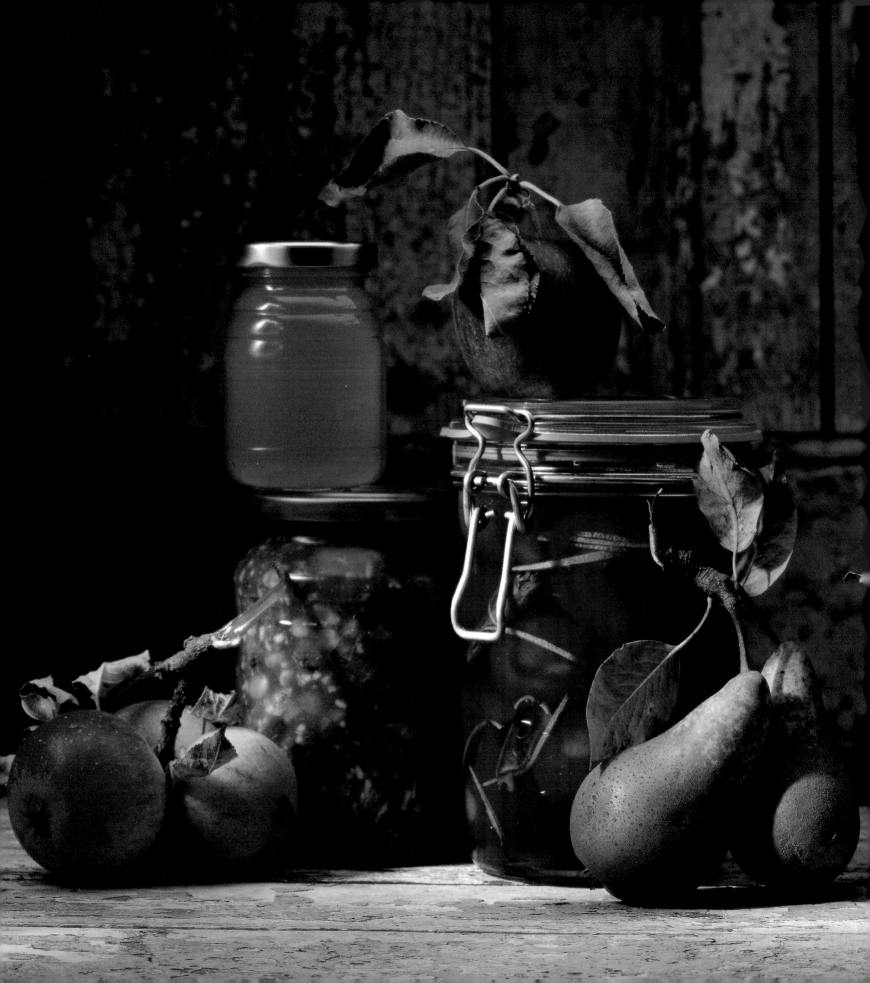

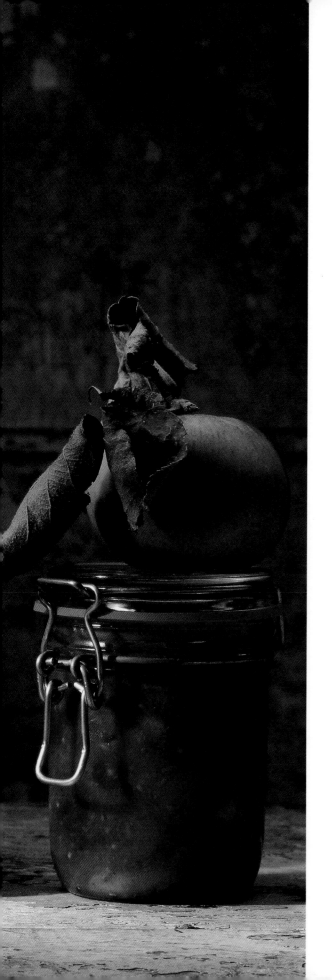

$\mathscr{A}$PPLES AND $\mathscr{P}$EARS

Traditionally, late summer and autumn, when the pear and apple crops were picked from laden trees in orchards and gardens, were the prime times for preserving. Now, not only do fewer people have their own apple and pear trees, but the fruits are imported in quantity all year round. Modern storage techniques mean that varieties such as Northern Spy and Winesap, very good cooking apples, are almost always available. This chapter also includes recipes for crab apples and quinces. These fruits grow wild and are difficult to find in the stores, as they only appear when in season.

Left, from left to right: Apple Honey; Apple, Citrus, and Whiskey Mincemeat; Mulled Pears; and Curried Apple and Carrot Chutney.

51

Apple and Cherry Jam

To overcome the problem of getting cherry jam to set because cherries have such a low pectin content, the cherries are sometimes cooked in red currant juice, which is high in natural pectin. Here, however, I have used the juice of cooking apples, as they are more abundant and less expensive than red currants, the flavor of the two fruits goes well together, and the jam looks attractive.

MAKES ABOUT 6 CUPS

1½ pounds tart, juicy cooking apples
3 pounds sour cooking cherries, pitted
2½ tablespoons lemon juice
6 cups warmed sugar (see page 7)

Slice the apples without peeling or coring them, then cook very gently in 2½ cups water in a large covered saucepan for about 30 minutes, stirring occasionally, until they are very soft. Pour the contents of this pan into a scalded jelly bag suspended over a bowl and leave to strain, undisturbed, in a cool place for 6–8 hours to make about 1¼ cups juice.

Gently simmer the apple juice, cherries, and lemon juice for about 30 minutes or until much of the water from the mixture has evaporated.

Remove the pan from the heat, stir in the sugar, then return to the heat and cook gently, stirring, until the sugar has dissolved. Raise the heat and boil vigorously for about 10 minutes, stirring as necessary, until setting point is reached (see page 17).

Remove from the heat and skim any scum from the surface with a slotted spoon. Pour into warm, clean, dry jars. Cover, seal, and process (see pages 12–13). Leave overnight to set. Store in a cool, dark, dry place.

Right: Apple and Cherry Puffs are discs of melt-in-your-mouth pastry filled with fruity jam.

Apple and Cherry Puffs

Made from soft cheese and without any water, the pastry in this recipe is meltingly light and short.

MAKES 12

½ cup unsalted butter, softened
4 ounces full-fat cream cheese
few drops of almond extract
1¼ cups all-purpose flour
Apple and Cherry Jam (see left)

In a bowl, beat the butter, cream cheese, and extract together, then gradually beat in the flour. Form into a ball, wrap in waxed paper or plastic wrap, and chill for 1 hour.

Preheat the oven to 400°F. On a lightly floured surface, roll out the pastry and cut into twelve 3-inch circles. Place a large teaspoonful of jam on each circle, fold the pastry in half, and press the edges together to seal. Transfer to a baking sheet and bake for about 15 minutes or until pale gold. Serve hot with crème fraîche or sour cream.

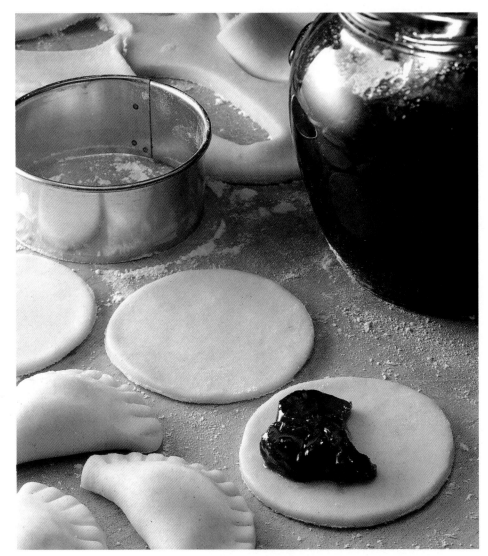

$\mathscr{A}$PPLES

Apple Honey

Adding apples and spices to an inexpensive honey transforms it into a luxurious-tasting spread. Either cooking or eating apples can be used, provided the latter are crisp, juicy, and not too sweet.

MAKES ABOUT 4 CUPS

3 pounds cooking or eating apples, chopped without peeling or coring
Per 2½ cups of juice:
1¾ cups sugar
⅓ cup clear honey
2-inch piece of cinnamon stick
3 whole cloves
small piece of fresh ginger

Put the apples and 3½ cups water in a large saucepan and cook for 20–30 minutes or until soft and pulpy, stirring occasionally. Pour the mixture into a scalded jelly bag suspended over a nonmetallic bowl and leave to strain, undisturbed, in a cool place for 8–12 hours.

Measure the apple juice, then pour it into the rinsed pan. Add the sugar, honey, and spices (tied in a cheesecloth bag), and heat gently, stirring, until the sugar has dissolved. Raise the heat and boil vigorously for about 4 minutes or until setting point is reached (see page 17).

Remove the pan from the heat, skim any scum from the surface of the honey with a slotted spoon, and discard the spice bag. Pour the honey into warm, clean, dry jars. Cover, seal, and process (see pages 12–13). Once set, this is ready to eat. Store in a cool, dark, dry place.

Serving Suggestion
Stir into thick yogurt or whipped cream; spoon onto pancakes or waffles; spread on bread, toast, or slices of plain cake.

Caramelized Apple Jam

Remove the pan from the heat once the caramel reaches the golden stage, as it can quickly turn bitter if it continues cooking.

MAKES ABOUT 5⅓ CUPS

5 pounds cooking apples
juice of 1 lemon
4½ cups sugar
¼ cup brandy or Calvados

Peel, core (see page 56), and dice the apples, then toss them in a bowl with the lemon juice to prevent discoloration.

Stir 2¼ cups sugar and ¼ cup water together in a large saucepan over low heat and bring slowly to a boil. Cook until golden brown, then quickly remove from the heat and immediately stir in the apples to mix well with the caramel (see below). The caramel will harden on contact with the apples but will melt again when heated. (Beware of scalding steam at this point.)

Add the remaining sugar, stirring until it has dissolved. Return the mixture to low heat and bring very slowly back to the boiling point, stirring frequently. Continue cooking for about 10–15 minutes or until the apples are very soft and some of the liquid

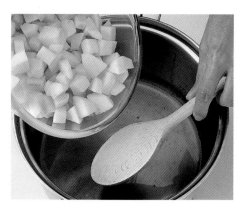

Adding the apples: As soon as the caramel has turned a light brown color, remove from the heat, stir in the diced apples, and combine well.

has boiled away. Press the apples through a nonmetallic sieve with a wooden spoon and return to the pan. If the purée is already very thick, boil for another minute; if it is thin, boil again until reduced and thickened.

Remove the pan from the heat and stir in the brandy. Spoon into warm, clean, dry jars. Cover, seal, and process (see pages 12–13). Leave overnight. Store in a cool, dark, dry place.

Apple Nectar

Cool glasses of Apple Nectar on a summer's day are just what the doctor ordered.

MAKES ABOUT 7½ CUPS

3 whole cloves
3 pounds cooking apples, peeled, quartered, and cored (about 2¼ pounds prepared)
2 cups sugar
juice of 1 lemon

Tie the cloves in a cheesecloth bag and put in a large saucepan with the apples and 1¼ cups water. Cover and cook gently for about 30 minutes, stirring occasionally, until the apples are tender. Discard the cheesecloth bag, then purée the apples in a blender or push the pulp through a nonmetallic sieve.

In a saucepan, gently heat the sugar in 2 cups water, stirring until dissolved. Raise the heat, add the lemon juice, and boil for 2 minutes. Stir in the purée and simmer for 10 minutes, stirring occasionally.

Adjust the heat if necessary so that the nectar is gently bubbling, and ladle into warm, clean, dry bottles. Cover, seal, and process (see pages 12–13). This will keep in a cool, dark, dry place for about 4 months. Shake the bottle before pouring.

Serving Suggestion
Serve chilled on its own or with cookies or cake; add to fruit salads.

Spiced Apple and Cider Butter

For this butter, use a well-flavored variety of eating apple for sweetness, and tart cooking apples, for kick. The amount of lemon juice needed will depend on the sweetness of the apples.

MAKES ABOUT 3⅓ CUPS

5 cups dry hard cider
1½ pounds cooking apples, peeled, cored, and sliced
1½ pounds well-flavored eating apples, peeled, cored, and sliced
grated zest and juice of 1 thin-skinned lemon
warmed sugar (see page 7)
½ teaspoon ground cinnamon
½ teaspoon freshly grated nutmeg

Pour the cider into a large saucepan and boil vigorously for 15 minutes or until reduced by half. Add the apples and lemon zest and juice, cover the pan, and cook for 20–30 minutes or until very soft and reduced to a purée, stirring occasionally to make sure the apples cook evenly and to break them up. Press the contents of the pan through a nonmetallic sieve into a bowl.

Weigh the purée and return it to the rinsed pan. Add ¾ cup plus 2 tablespoons sugar for every 1½ cups purée, the cinnamon, and nutmeg and stir over low heat until the sugar has dissolved. Then boil gently for 35–45 minutes, stirring occasionally and then more frequently, until the stirring is constant and the mixture has the consistency of sour cream.

Spoon into warm, clean, dry jars. Cover, seal, and process (see pages 12–13). Store the butter in a cool, dark, dry place for a few days before eating.

Serving Suggestions
Use as a base for thickly sliced apples in an apple tart.

Spiced Apple and Orange Jelly

I make this jelly in winter partly because no seasonal ingredients are called for and partly because its warm, spicy, tangy flavor seems more appropriate for winter days and winter meals.

MAKES ABOUT 3⅓ CUPS

1½ pounds cooking apples, chopped without peeling and coring
4 large oranges, chopped with peel
1 large lemon, chopped with peel
1 cinnamon stick
1-ounce piece of unpeeled fresh ginger, sliced
warmed sugar (see page 7)

Put all the ingredients except the sugar in a large saucepan and add 7½ cups water. Bring to a boil, then cover and simmer gently, stirring occasionally, for about 1 hour or until the fruit is soft.

Pour the contents of the pan into a scalded jelly bag suspended over a nonmetallic bowl and leave to strain, undisturbed, in a cool place for 8–12 hours.

Measure the juice and pour it back into the rinsed pan. Add 2¼ cups sugar for every 2½ cups juice and heat gently, stirring, until the sugar has dissolved, then boil vigorously for about 10 minutes or until setting point is reached (see page 17).

Remove the pan from the heat and skim off any scum with a slotted spoon. Pour into warm, clean, dry jars. Cover, seal, and process (see pages 12–13). Leave overnight to set. Store in a cool, dark, dry place.

Variation: *Spiced Apple Jelly*
Use 1½ pounds cooking apples, 2 sliced lemons, 1 ounce sliced fresh ginger, 1 cinnamon stick, ½ teaspoon whole cloves, ¾ cup white wine vinegar, and 7½ cups water. Follow the method above.

Apple, Citrus, and Whiskey Mincemeat

This is a moist, tangy, spicy mincemeat.

MAKES 5⅓ CUPS

1¼ pounds cooking apples, peeled, cored, and chopped
1 tablespoon butter
⅔ cup dried apricot halves, chopped
1⅓ cups golden raisins
1⅓ cups seedless raisins
1¼ cups dark raw sugar
¾ cup currants
⅔ cup mixed candied peel
¾ cup hazelnuts, skinned and coarsely chopped
¾ cup blanched almonds, coarsely chopped
grated zest and juice of 1 orange
grated zest and juice of 1 lemon
1 teaspoon ground cinnamon
½ teaspoon ground ginger
½ teaspoon freshly grated nutmeg
pinch of ground cloves
½ cup vegetarian or beef suet
⅔ cup whiskey

Gently cook the apples with ¼ cup water and the butter in a large covered saucepan for about 20 minutes or until soft and pulpy. Remove the lid, raise the heat, and cook, stirring, for about 10 minutes or until almost all the liquid has evaporated. Leave to cool.

Stir the remaining ingredients together in a large nonmetallic bowl. Stir in the apples. Cover and leave overnight in a cool place.

The next day, give the mincemeat a good stir, then pack it firmly into clean, dry jars, taking care not to trap any air bubbles. Cover, seal, and process (see pages 12–13). Store in a cool, dark, dry place for at least 6 weeks before using.

Serving Suggestion
Serve with poached orange slices or use as a filling for pies and tarts.

*A*PPLES

Minted Apple Relish

Vary the flavor of this relish by using different types of mint. Spearmint is the most common garden mint, but you can also try apple, lemon, pineapple, or ginger mint.

MAKES ABOUT ⅔ CUP

8 ounces onions, sliced
2 teaspoons dry English mustard
1 teaspoon black peppercorns
1 cinnamon stick, broken in half
¼ teaspoon ground mace
1 teaspoon sea salt
1¼ cups sugar
1¼ cups Spiced Vinegar (see page 139)
1½ pounds cooking apples, peeled, cored, and thinly sliced
½ ounce fresh mint, finely chopped

Put all the ingredients except the apples and mint in a large saucepan and heat gently, stirring, until the sugar has dissolved. Bring to a boil, then simmer gently for 10 minutes. Stir in the apples and continue cooking for another 10 minutes or until the apples are tender but still retain their shape.

Remove the mixture from the heat and leave to cool. Remove the cinnamon stick and pack the relish into warm clean, dry jars, sprinkling mint between the layers and taking care not to trap any air pockets. Cover with acid-proof lids, seal, and process (see pages 12–13). Store in a cool, dark, dry place for 1 month before eating.

Serving Suggestion
Use as a stuffing for a boned leg or shoulder of lamb; stir into freshly cooked new potatoes and leave to cool, then serve as a salad; serve with smoked pork loin or smoked chicken.

Curried Apple and Carrot Chutney

Fresh horseradish enlivens this chutney.

MAKES ABOUT 3⅓ CUPS

1¼ pounds cooking apples, peeled, cored, and chopped
9 ounces carrots, thinly sliced lengthwise
1 onion, sliced
⅔ cup raisins
4 ounces fresh horseradish, grated
1 tablespoon curry powder
1 tablespoon ground ginger
1 teaspoon mustard seeds
1¼ cups cider vinegar
1¼ cups light brown sugar
2 teaspoons sea salt

Stir all the ingredients together in a large saucepan and heat gently, stirring constantly, until the sugar has dissolved. Bring to a boil, then simmer, stirring frequently, for about 30–45 minutes or until the ingredients are tender, the chutney is thick, and there is no free liquid.

Spoon into warm, clean, dry jars, taking care not to trap any air bubbles. Cover with acid-proof lids, seal, and process (see pages 12–13). Store in a cool, dark, dry place for 2 months before eating.

Serving Suggestion
Serve as an accompaniment to spicy northern Indian food.

Below: If you grow your own apples and mint, Minted Apple Relish is inexpensive to make.

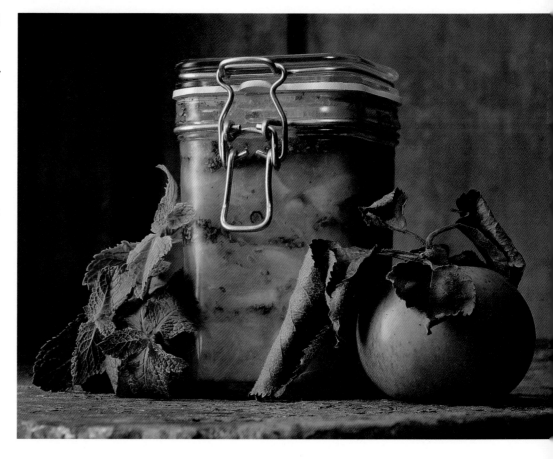

Uncooked Apple Chutney

This simple chutney couldn't be easier or quicker to make.

MAKES ABOUT 3 CUPS

1⅓ cups golden raisins
1 tablespoon chopped fresh ginger
3 tablespoons brown mustard seeds
1¼ cups demerara or raw sugar
2 teaspoons sea salt
1¼ cups cider vinegar
1½ pounds cooking apples, peeled, cored (see below), and coarsely chopped
8 ounces onions, very finely chopped
2 garlic cloves, very finely chopped (optional)

Stir the raisins, ginger, mustard seeds, sugar, salt, and vinegar together in a nonmetallic bowl until the sugar has dissolved.

Stir in the apples, onion and garlic if using. Cover and leave in a cool place for 1 week, stirring once every day.

Spoon the chutney into clean, dry jars, taking care not to trap any air bubbles. Cover with acid-proof lids, seal, and process (see pages 12–13). This chutney is now ready to eat. Store in a cool, dark, dry

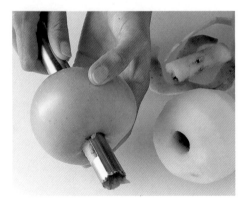

Coring apples: An apple corer is the quickest, easiest, and most efficient way of removing the cores from apples and other fruits.

place. Keep the chutney tightly covered to make sure it doesn't dry out.

Serving Suggestion
Stir into the skimmed pan juices from roast pork and serve with the meat. It is also good with a picnic lunch of hard cheese and crusty bread.

Crab Apple and Clove Jelly

Crab apples are too hard and astringent to eat raw and too small to peel and core. Making a jelly is therefore an ideal way of using them. Cloves bring out the warm, spicy note in their flavor.

MAKES 4⅔–5⅓ CUPS

5½ pounds crab apples
6 whole cloves
warmed sugar (see page 7)

Chop the crab apples without peeling or coring them and put them into a large saucepan with the cloves and 7½ cups water. Bring to a boil, then cover and simmer for about 1¼ hours, stirring occasionally, until soft and pulpy.

Pour the contents of the pan into a scalded jelly bag suspended over a large nonmetallic bowl and leave to strain, undisturbed, in a cool place for 8–12 hours. Measure the juice and pour into the rinsed pan. Add 2¼ cups sugar for every 2½ cups juice and heat gently, stirring, until the sugar has dissolved. Raise the heat and boil vigorously for about 10 minutes or until setting point is reached (see page 17). Remove the mixture from the heat and skim the scum from the surface with a slotted spoon. Pour the jelly into warm, clean, dry jars. Cover, seal, and process (see pages 12–13). Leave overnight to set. Store in a cool, dark, dry place.

Mulled Pears

Use a soft, fruity wine such as a Loire red like Chinon or a Beaujolais rather than more robust types such as young Cabernet Sauvignon wines.

MAKES ABOUT 1¾ QUARTS

3 pounds small underripe pears, such as Bosc
whole cloves
3-inch piece cinnamon stick, broken into pieces
2 blades of mace
3-inch piece of fresh ginger, chopped
zest of 1 small lemon, cut into thin strips
1¼ cups sugar
about 2¼ cups red wine

Preheat the oven to 250°F.

Carefully peel the pears, leaving the stems intact. Stud each pear with a clove, then divide them between three 1-pint jars. Distribute the spices, ginger, lemon zest, sugar, and wine between the jars, making sure the pears are covered with liquid. Cover but do not seal the jars. Put in the oven for 3 hours. Remove and seal the jars (see pages 12–13). Once cool, store in a cool, dark, dry place.

Variation: *Cherries in Red Wine*
Gently heat 1¼ cups sugar in 2½ cups red wine until dissolved, then add 2 fresh bay leaves and simmer for 10 minutes or until syrupy. Add 2 pounds cherries and cook gently until they are tender. Pour the cherries and syrup into a clean, warm, dry jar, discarding the bay leaves. Cover and seal. Makes about 1½ quarts.

Serving Suggestion
Serve very cold with crème caramel or rice pudding; use in clafoutis or tarts (see opposite); or serve with roast duck, venison, or squab, deglazing the cooking juices with some of the syrup and lemon juice.

Mulled Pear Tart

SERVES 4–6

1½ cups all-purpose flour
pinch of salt
½ cup confectioners' sugar, sifted
½ cup unsalted butter, softened
1 large egg yolk
1 tablespoon cold water
1 cup half-and-half
1 vanilla bean
3 extra-large egg yolks
⅓ cup granulated sugar
2 tablespoons all-purpose flour mixed with
    2 tablespoons cornstarch
1 tablespoon unsalted butter, diced
about ⅔ cup juice from the Mulled Pears
10 Mulled Pears (see page 56), halved

Sift the flour and salt onto a work surface and make a well in the center. Put the confectioners' sugar, butter, 1 egg yolk, and water into the well. Pinch together into a paste, then draw in the flour to form a ball. Put on a plate, cover, and chill for 2 hours.

Roll out the pastry and use to line a loose-bottomed 9-inch fluted tart pan, pressing the pastry well into the sides and base. Run the rolling pin over the top to cut off excess pastry. Chill for 20 minutes.

Meanwhile, preheat the oven to 400°F. Prick the base of the pastry shell, line with waxed paper, and weight down with dried beans or pie weights. Bake for about 12 minutes, then lower the oven temperature to 375°F. Remove the paper and beans from the pastry shell and bake for another 8–10 minutes or until the pastry is pale gold. Leave to cool on a wire rack.

To make the crème pâtissière, gently heat the half-and-half and the vanilla bean to simmering, remove from the heat, cover, and leave for 30 minutes. Whisk the egg yolks and sugar in a bowl until thick. Sift the flour and cornstarch into the egg mixture and beat. Boil the milk mixture and strain into the egg mixture, whisking constantly.

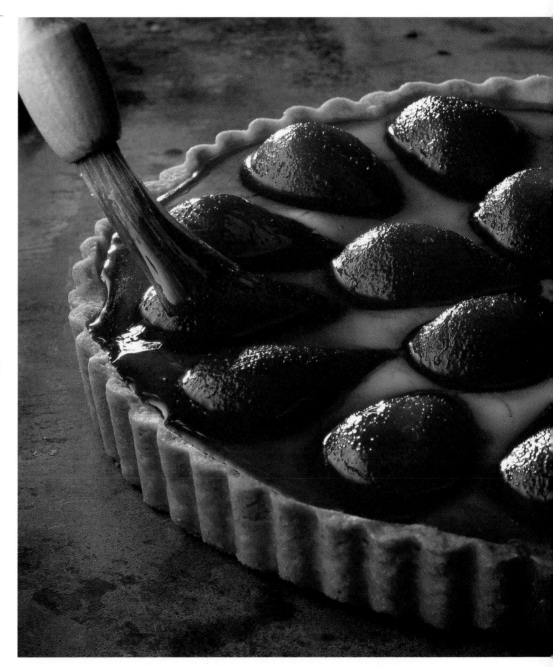

Return the mixture to the pan and bring to a boil, whisking. Simmer for 2–3 minutes. Remove the pan from the heat, stir in the butter, and pour the mixture into a bowl. Leave to cool, stirring occasionally, then cover and chill in the refrigerator.

Above: Meltingly spicy Mulled Pear Tart.

Boil the juice from the pears until syrupy and leave to cool. Fill the pastry shell with the crème pâtissière. Lay the pears on top and brush with the syrupy liquid.

Pear Chutney

When making this extremely simple recipe, I sometimes use chopped pitted prunes or currants instead of raisins or add chopped onions or some allspice.

MAKES 4⅔–5⅓ CUPS

3 pounds firm-ripe pears, cored and chopped but not peeled
2 large garlic cloves, finely chopped
2 teaspoons sea salt
1–2 teaspoons cayenne pepper, to taste
2 teaspoons freshly ground coriander
2 tablespoons chopped fresh ginger
1⅓ cups plump raisins
½ cup white wine vinegar
½ cup lime juice
1 cup warmed light brown sugar (see page 7)

Put all the ingredients except the sugar in a large saucepan, cover, and simmer for 15 minutes, stirring occasionally, until the pears are soft.

Add the warmed sugar and stir until dissolved, then bring the mixture to a boil. The mixture should be a thick, soft purée

with no free liquid; if it seems too thick, add about ½ cup water and boil again for about 10 minutes, stirring, until the right consistency is reached.

Ladle into warm, clean, dry jars, taking care not to trap any air bubbles. Cover with acid-proof lids, seal, and process (see pages 12–13). Store in a cool, dark, dry place for at least 1–2 months before eating.

Pear and Pineapple Conserve

Reserve the juices that come from the pineapple when you are preparing it to add to the cooking liquid.

MAKES 3⅓ CUPS

1½ pounds large pineapple, peeled, cored, and finely chopped to make 1 pound flesh
2¼ pounds firm-ripe pears, peeled, cored, and thinly sliced
commercial liquid pectin or 1 cup pectin extract (see page 7)
2¼ cups warmed sugar (see page 7)

Gently cook the pineapple in 1 cup water and the reserved pineapple juices in a small covered saucepan for 35–40 minutes or until it is just tender. Add the pears and pectin extract and cook gently for another 20–25 minutes, covered, until both fruits are tender (if using commercial pectin, follow the manufacturer's directions).

Over low heat, add the sugar and stir until it has dissolved, then boil vigorously, without stirring, for 20–30 minutes or until thickened and a light set is reached.

Ladle into warm, clean, dry jars. Cover, seal, and process (see pages 12–13). Leave overnight. Store in a cool, dark, dry place.

Spiced Pears

This puts flavorless pears to good use.

MAKES 5 CUPS

3 pounds firm pears, peeled
1 teaspoon allspice berries
1-inch piece of fresh ginger, sliced
1 teaspoon whole cloves
2 cinnamon sticks
1¼ cups sugar
2 cups white wine vinegar

Halve or quarter the pears. Remove the cores and put the pears in a large saucepan with enough water just to cover them. Bring to a boil, then simmer for 5 minutes.

Drain the pears, reserving the liquid. Add water to the liquid to make 2 cups, then pour back into the pan. Add the remaining ingredients except the pears and cook over low heat, stirring, until the sugar has dissolved, then simmer for 5 minutes.

Add the pears to the pan and simmer for 20–30 minutes or until they are tender and translucent but still hold their shape.

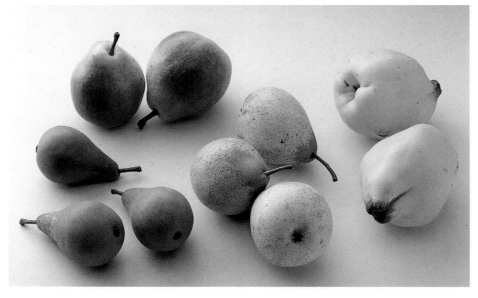

Left, clockwise from right: Quinces, Comice pears, Conference pears, and Bartlett pears.

Quinces and Crab Apples

Use a slotted spoon to transfer the pears to a warm, clean, dry jar, then pour in the liquid and spices. Cover with an acid-proof lid, seal, and process (see pages 12–13). Store in a cool, dark, dry place for at least 1 month before eating.

Serving Suggestion
Serve with cold roast pork; use the spiced vinegar to make salad dressings.

Quince Spread

The wonderful flavor of the sweetened cooked fruit (which is inedible raw) will permeate fruits cooked with it, so if you do not have enough quinces, combine them with apples and a chopped slice of orange. Use quinces when they are yellow all over.

MAKES ABOUT 4 CUPS

3 pounds quinces
warmed sugar (see page 7)

Wash the gray off the quinces, then chop the fruit, including the skins and cores. Put into a large saucepan, just cover with water, and simmer gently for 30–45 minutes or until the fruit is tender.

Pour the contents of the pan into a nonmetallic sieve over a nonmetallic bowl and press through with a wooden spoon. Measure the purée and return to the rinsed-out pan. Add 2¼ cups sugar for each 2½ cups purée and heat gently, stirring, until the sugar has dissolved. Bring the mixture to a boil, then continue to boil, stirring frequently, for 45–55 minutes or until it is so thick that the spoon leaves a clean line when drawn through it.

Spoon into warm, clean, dry jars or lightly oiled molds, cover with waxed paper, seal, and process (see pages 12–13). Store in a cool, dark, dry place for at least 2–3 months before eating.

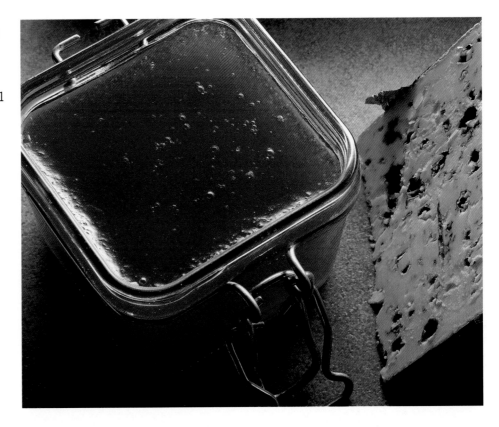

Spiced Crab Apples

This recipe makes a refreshing change from the more traditional crab apple jelly or crab apple butter.

MAKES ABOUT 6 CUPS

3 pounds crab apples, unpeeled
2 strips lemon rind
generous 1 cup granulated sugar
1 cup white wine vinegar
1½-inch piece cinnamon stick
1 clove
2 black peppercorns

Put the crab apples in a large saucepan. Add 2 cups water and the lemon rind. Bring to a boil, then simmer gently for about 6 minutes or until the fruit is almost tender.

Strain the crab apples through a colander, reserving the liquid.

Above: This glowing Quince Spread is delicious eaten with Danish Blue or Stilton cheese.

Put the sugar, 2 cups of the reserved liquid, and the vinegar into a clean saucepan.

Tie the spices in a piece of cheesecloth and add to the pan. Heat gently, stirring, until the sugar has dissolved. Bring to a boil and boil for 1 minute.

Add the crab apples and simmer very gently, taking care the fruit doesn't start to break up, for 30–40 minutes or until the liquid has reduced to coating consistency. Remove from the heat and discard the cheesecloth bag.

Using a slotted spoon, transfer the apples to warm, clean, dry jars. Fill the jars with the syrup. Cover, seal, and process (see pages 12–13). Store in a cool, dark, dry place for 2 months before eating, or up to 1 year.

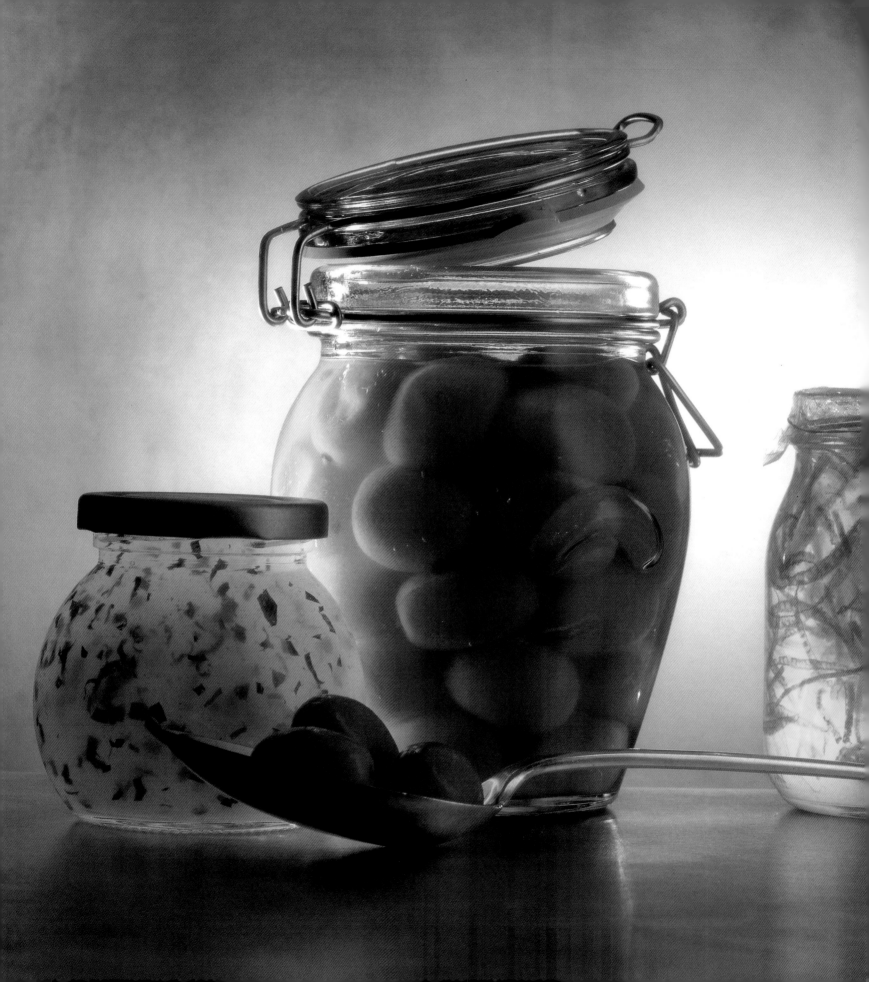

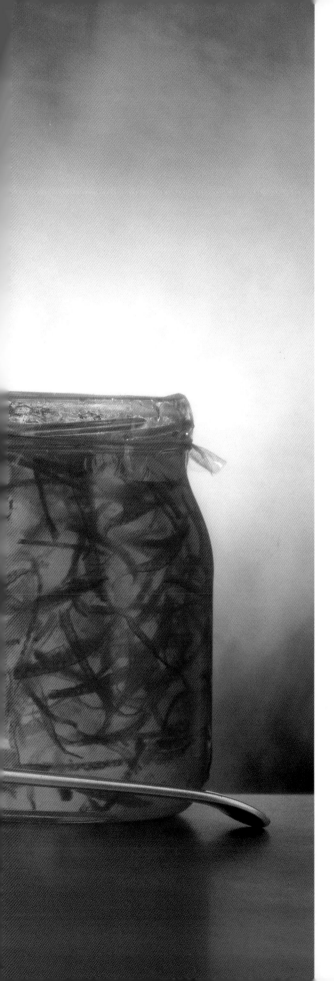

CITRUS FRUITS

Marmalade is the preserve most obviously associated with citrus fruits and possibly the only one that many people will think of, at least immediately. Indeed, all citrus fruits, not just oranges, are used for marmalades because their sharp flavors, especially when the peel is included, seem to be just what is needed for breakfast. Citrus peels harden when cooked with sugar, so they must first be completely softened before the sugar is added to the mixture. These fruits have a high pectin content, so they set easily and are natural candidates for making jams and jellies. Their fresh, tangy flavor makes them ideal for a whole host of other preserves, varying from Kumquats or Tangerines in Vodka and Cointreau (see page 72) to chutneys, Moroccan Preserved Lemons (see page 75), Indian Sweet-Sour Lime Pickle (see page 77), and, typically, English fruit curds. Citrus peel can also be candied for use in baking or to eat with coffee after dinner.

Left, from left to right: Orange and Tarragon Jelly, Kumquats in Vodka and Cointreau, and Seville Orange Marmalade.

Oxford Marmalade

The characteristic dark color and deep flavor of traditional Oxford marmalade is the result of long boiling before the sugar is added.

MAKES ABOUT 6⅔ CUPS

1½ pounds Seville oranges
1¾ quarts boiling water
7 cups warmed sugar (see page 7)

Peel the oranges and cut the peel into chunky strips. Chop the flesh, reserving the seeds. Put the flesh and peel strips into a large nonmetallic bowl and the seeds into a small one. Pour 1¼ cups of the boiling water into the small bowl with the seeds and the remainder into the large bowl. Cover both bowls and leave overnight.

Pour the seeds into a nonmetallic sieve placed over the large bowl, using their water to wash off the soft, clear jelly surrounding them. If necessary, ladle some of the water from the large bowl over the seeds to rinse them again; discard the seeds.

Pour the contents of the large bowl into a large saucepan, bring to a boil, and simmer

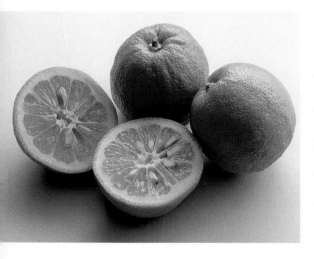

Above: Seville oranges from Spain are used for making many traditional marmalades.

gently for 2–2½ hours, stirring occasionally, until the peel is very soft – the longer the boiling, the darker the marmalade will be. Add more water during boiling if necessary.

Over low heat, stir in the warmed sugar until it has dissolved. Boil gently until the desired color is reached, then raise the heat and boil vigorously for another 15–20 minutes, stirring as necessary, until setting point is reached (see page 17).

Remove the pan from the heat and skim the scum from the marmalade's surface with a slotted spoon. Leave to stand for 10–15 minutes, then stir and ladle into warm, clean, dry jars. Cover, seal, and process (see pages 12–13). Leave overnight to set. Store in a cool, dark, dry place.

Leisurely Marmalade

This marmalade is made at a leisurely pace over three days – hence its name.

MAKES ABOUT 3⅔ CUPS

6 large sweet oranges
½ large lemon
warmed sugar (see page 7)

Remove the stem ends from the fruit and discard. Slice the fruit and leave to soak in a large covered saucepan with 2¼ cups water for one day.

The next day, bring the mixture to a boil, then simmer gently, stirring occasionally, for 25–50 minutes or so, depending how soft you want the peel to be. Remove from the heat and leave to cool, then cover and leave for another day.

Weigh the fruit and juice and return to the pan with 3⅓ cups warmed sugar for every 1 pound of fruit and juice. Stir to dissolve the sugar, then bring the mixture to a boil and boil vigorously, stirring as necessary, for about 1 hour or until setting point is reached (see page 17).

Remove from the heat and skim the scum from the surface with a slotted spoon. Leave to stand for 10–15 minutes. Stir and ladle into warm, clean, dry jars. Cover, seal, and process (see pages 12–13). Leave overnight to set. Store in a cool, dark, dry place.

Ginger and Apple Marmalade

Ground and preserved ginger add warmth to this marmalade, making it particularly appropriate for winter.

MAKES ABOUT 6⅔ CUPS

8 ounces Seville oranges
1½ pounds cooking apples, peeled, cored, and chopped
8¼ cups warmed sugar (see page 7)
2 teaspoons ground ginger
½ cup preserved ginger in syrup, diced

Peel the oranges and finely chop the peel. Coarsely chop the orange flesh, removing and reserving the membranes, pith, and seeds. Tie the membranes, pith, and seeds in a cheesecloth bag with a long length of string. Put the chopped orange, peel, juice, and 1½ quarts water in a pan, and tie the cheesecloth bag on the pan handle so that the bag is suspended in the mixture. Bring to a boil, then simmer for 1–1½ hours, stirring occasionally, until the peel is soft and the contents of the pan are reduced by half.

Remove the pan from the heat. Scoop out the cheesecloth bag with a slotted spoon and press the bag firmly with the back of a metal spoon so that the juices run back into the pan. Discard the bag.

Meanwhile, simmer the apples in ⅔ cup water for about 8 minutes or until pulpy.

Add the apple pulp, sugar, ground ginger, and preserved ginger to the oranges and stir until the sugar has dissolved. Raise the heat

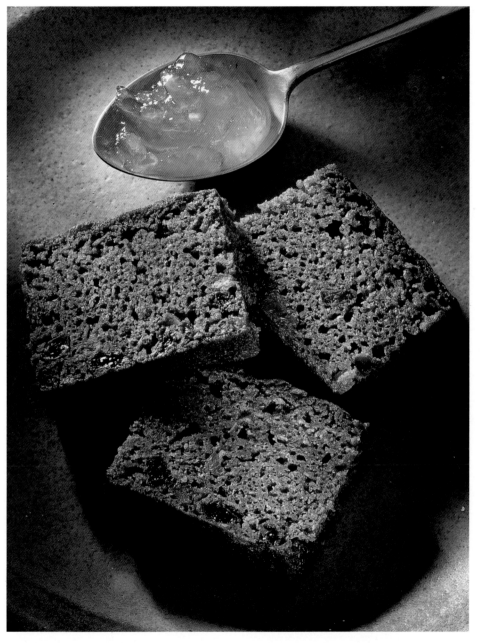

Marmalade Gingerbread

Instead of adding corn syrup and molasses to gingerbread, I tried adding marmalade and this is now the only way I make such cakes. Marmalades I have used are Seville Orange (see pages 18–19), Pineapple and Orange (see page 65), Tangerine (see page 70), and Peach (see page 101), each one giving its own unique character to the gingerbread. However, ordinary store-bought marmalades will also produce a good result. This gingerbread is best kept for a couple of days before being eaten.

MAKES AN 8- OR 9-INCH ROUND CAKE

1 cup butter, diced
1¼ cups dark brown sugar
1¼ cups milk
⅔ cup marmalade (see above)
3 cups self-rising flour
1½–2 tablespoons ground ginger
2 teaspoons baking soda
2 teaspoons ground cinnamon
1 teaspoon freshly grated nutmeg
2 extra-large eggs, beaten
7 pieces preserved ginger in syrup, chopped
⅔ cup plump raisins

Preheat the oven to 310°F. Butter an 8- or 9-inch round cake pan and line the base with waxed paper.

In a large saucepan, gently heat together the butter, sugar, milk, and marmalade, stirring occasionally, until the butter and sugar have melted. Remove from the heat and leave to cool. Stir together the flour, ginger, baking soda, cinnamon, and nutmeg and form a well in the center. Slowly pour in the marmalade mixture, stirring the dry ingredients into the liquid to make a smooth batter; add the eggs toward the end. Stir in the chopped ginger and raisins. Pour the mixture into the cake pan and bake for about 1½ hours or until risen and firm to the touch in the center. Leave to cool in the pan. Store in an airtight container.

and boil vigorously for about 25 minutes, stirring as necessary, until setting point is reached (see page 17).

Remove the pan from the heat and skim the scum from the surface with a slotted spoon. Leave to stand for 10–15 minutes, stir to distribute the peel and ginger, and

Above: Marmalade Gingerbread is a moist cake that will keep well in an airtight container.

ladle into warm, clean, dry jars. Cover, seal, and process (see pages 12–13). Leave the marmalade overnight to set. Store in a cool, dark, dry place.

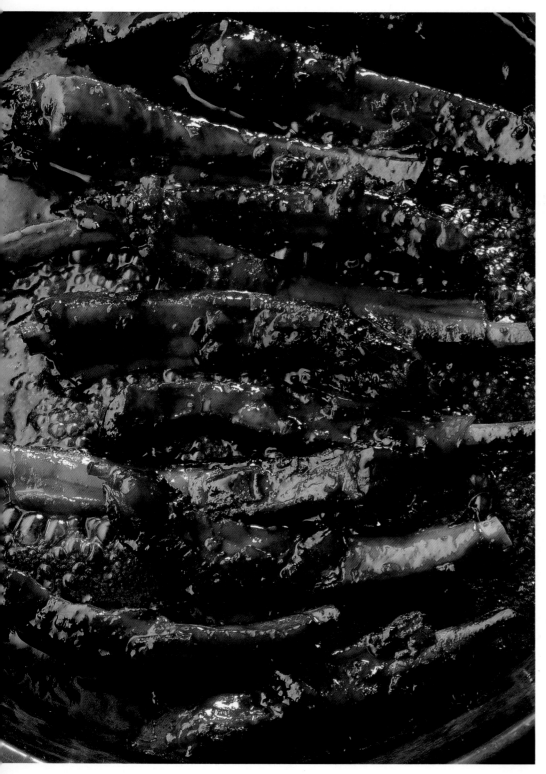

Glazed Spare Ribs

These ribs are great for family dinners or informal meals. The best marmalades to use are Ginger and Apple Marmalade (see page 62), Grapefruit, Orange, and Lemon Marmalade (see page 65) and Seville Orange Marmalade (see pages 18–19).

SERVES 4

½ cup marmalade (see above)
2 tablespoons clear honey
2 garlic cloves, crushed
1¼ cups dry hard cider
½ cup soy sauce
3 tablespoons lime juice
freshly ground black pepper
4 pounds pork spare ribs
lime wedges to garnish

Place all the ingredients except the pork and lime wedges in a saucepan and gently heat together until blended, stirring as necessary. Remove from the heat and leave to cool.

Divide the pork into individual ribs if necessary and trim away the excess fat. Put the ribs in a large nonmetallic dish, add the cold marmalade mixture, cover, and leave in the refrigerator for about 12 hours, turning the ribs occasionally.

Preheat the oven to 375°F. Transfer the ribs and marmalade mixture to a roasting pan about 20 minutes before cooking. Cover the roasting pan with aluminum foil and bake the ribs for 1 hour. Uncover the pan and bake for another hour, basting occasionally, until the ribs are cooked through and the juices run clear if the meat is pierced with the tip of a knife.

Place the roasting pan on the stove and cook over high heat for 3–7 minutes, stirring and turning the ribs until they are coated with a sticky glaze. Serve garnished with lime wedges.

Left: Marmalade adds a delicious tang to the Chinese-style marinade for Glazed Spare Ribs.

Oranges

Grapefruit, Orange, and Lemon Marmalade

This marmalade contains fruits that are available throughout the year.

MAKES ABOUT 6⅔ CUPS

8 ounces sweet oranges
2 lemons
8 ounces grapefruit
7 cups warmed sugar (see page 7)

Cut the oranges and lemons in half, squeeze out the juice, and pour into a large saucepan; reserve the seeds and peel. Remove the membranes from the orange and lemon peel and also any excessive amount of pith on any of the peel. Score the grapefruit peel into quarters then remove it and reserve. Chop the grapefruit flesh, reserving the seeds, coarse membranes, and pith. Add the flesh to the pan. Tie all the membranes, pith, and seeds in a cheesecloth bag with a long length of string. Tie the end of the string to the pan handle so that the bag is suspended in the mixture.

Chop all the peel and add to the pan with 7½ cups water. Bring the mixture to a boil, then simmer gently for about 2 hours or until the peel is tender and the contents of the pan reduced by about half.

Using a slotted spoon, scoop out the cheesecloth bag and press the bag with the back of a metal spoon so that the juice runs back into the pan. Discard the bag.

Over low heat, stir in the warmed sugar until it has dissolved. Raise the heat and boil vigorously for about 15 minutes, stirring as necessary, until setting point is reached (see page 17).

Remove from the heat. Skim any scum from the surface with a slotted spoon. Leave to stand for 10–15 minutes, then stir and ladle into warm, clean, dry jars. Cover, seal, and process (see pages 12–13). Leave overnight to set. Store in a cool, dark, dry place.

Pineapple and Orange Marmalade

MAKES ABOUT 4 CUPS

2 sweet oranges, ends removed and thinly sliced
1 lemon, ends removed and thinly sliced
1½ pounds pineapple, peeled, cored, and chopped to produce 1 pound flesh
4½ cups warmed sugar (see page 7)

Cut the orange and lemon slices into quarters or eighths and reserve the seeds. Tie the seeds in a cheesecloth bag with a long length of string and put the bag into a large saucepan with the orange and lemon pieces and the pineapple, tying the end of the string to the handle so that the bag is suspended in the pan. Just cover with water and bring to a boil, then cover the pan and simmer for 35–45 minutes or until the fruit and peel are tender.

Scoop out the cheesecloth bag with a slotted spoon and press the bag firmly with the back of a metal spoon so that the juices run back into the pan. Discard the bag.

Over low heat, stir in the sugar until it has dissolved, then raise the heat and boil for 10–15 minutes, stirring as necessary, until setting point is reached (see page 17).

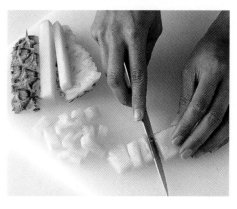

Preparing pineapples: Remove the core and all the eyes from the pineapple before cutting the flesh into evenly-sized pieces.

Remove from the heat and skim the scum from the surface with a slotted spoon. Leave to stand for 10–15 minutes, then stir and ladle into warm, clean, dry jars. Cover, seal, and process (see pages 12–13). Leave overnight to set. Store the marmalade in a cool, dark, dry place.

Rhubarb and Orange Chutney

Dried figs give this chutney an unusual taste.

MAKES ABOUT 5⅓ CUPS

1 pound rhubarb, finely chopped
8 ounces onions, finely chopped
grated zest and juice of 1 orange
1 cup dried figs, very finely chopped
⅓ cup plump raisins
2¼ cups sugar
1¾ cups Spiced Vinegar (see page 139)
1½ teaspoons brown mustard seeds
½–¾ teaspoon allspice berries
1½ teaspoons black peppercorns, crushed

Put all the ingredients except the spices in a large saucepan. Tie the spices in a cheesecloth bag with a long length of string and add to the pan, tying the string to the handle so that the bag is suspended in the mixture. Heat gently, stirring, until the sugar has dissolved. Bring the mixture to a boil, then simmer gently, stirring occasionally, for 1 hour or until the chutney is thick and no free liquid is visible.

Scoop out the cheesecloth bag with a slotted spoon and press the bag firmly with the back of a metal spoon so that the juices run back into the pan. Discard the bag. Ladle the chutney into warm, clean, dry jars; do not trap any air bubbles. Cover with acid-proof lids, seal, and process (see pages 12–13). Store in a cool, dark, dry place for 2 months before eating.

Pickled Orange Wedges

I like to have a jar of these wedges in the pantry. This is such an easy recipe to make, when I have some suitable oranges, I usually pickle a few this way.

MAKES 4 CUPS

4 plump thin-skinned oranges
2¼ cups sugar
12 whole cloves
½-ounce piece of fresh ginger, chopped
3-inch piece cinnamon stick
2 tablespoons allspice berries
2½ cups white wine vinegar

Cut each orange into 8–12 segments; discard the seeds. Put the segments into a flameproof casserole, just cover with water, and simmer for 45–60 minutes or until the orange peels are tender, but be careful not to overcook the fruit.

Meanwhile, gently heat the sugar, cloves, ginger, cinnamon stick, and allspice berries in the vinegar, stirring, until the sugar has dissolved. Raise the heat and bring the mixture to a boil, then simmer for 10 minutes, stirring as necessary.

Preheat the oven to 275°F.

Strain off and discard the liquid from the casserole, then replace it with the hot vinegar. Cover the casserole and put it in the oven for about 1 hour or until the orange peels are translucent.

Using a slotted spoon, transfer the oranges to warm, clean, dry jars and keep warm in the turned-off oven.

Boil the vinegar for about 10 minutes, until it is beginning to thicken, then pour over the oranges to cover completely. Rotate the jars to expel any air bubbles. Distribute the spices between the jars, breaking the cinnamon as necessary. Cover with acid-proof lids, seal, and process (see pages 12–13). Store in a cool, dark, dry place for 2 months before eating.

Serving Suggestion

Serve with hot or cold roast pork, ham, or game; broiled, grilled, or roast duck.

Honey-Spiced Pickled Oranges

Honey adds a special flavor that combines well with the orange, spices, and white wine vinegar in this pickle.

MAKES ABOUT 4 CUPS

6 oranges, cut into ¼-inch slices
1 cinnamon stick
1 teaspoon coriander seeds
1 teaspoon cardamom seeds
½ teaspoon black peppercorns, crushed
½ teaspoon whole cloves
1 cup sugar
¾ cup clear honey
1¼ cups white wine vinegar

Put the orange slices in a large saucepan and cover them with water. Cover the pan and bring to a boil, then simmer for 30 minutes. Drain the orange slices well.

Heat the cinnamon stick, coriander seeds, and cardamom seeds in a dry heavy skillet until they are fragrant, moving them gently around the pan to prevent them from burning. Remove from the heat, then lightly crush the seeds using a mortar and pestle or a coffee or spice grinder. Put all the spices, including the peppercorns and cloves, in a pan. Add the sugar, honey, and vinegar and heat gently, stirring, until the sugar has dissolved. Raise the heat and bring to a boil, then simmer for 10 minutes.

Add the orange slices and return the mixture to a boil, then cover and simmer for about 20 minutes or until the orange slices are translucent. Using a slotted spoon, transfer the slices to warm, clean, dry jars. Add the spices and cover with the vinegar.

Cover the jars immediately with acid-proof lids, seal, and process (see pages 12–13). Store in a cool, dark, dry place for at least 1 month before eating.

Spiced Candied Orange Peel

Any homemade candied peel is far better to eat than all but the most special, and costly, store-bought peels, and giving your peel a spicy flavor makes it stand out even more. Leaving the peel in large pieces keeps it deliciously moist.

6 oranges, lemons, grapefruit, or limes,
  or a mixture
1¾ cups sugar
6 whole cloves
1 cinnamon stick

Halve or quarter the fruit and remove the peels in single pieces. Simmer the peels in a little water for 1–2 hours, stirring occasionally, until tender. Change the water 2 or 3 times when cooking grapefruit peel. Drain and reserve the water and add more water to make 1¼ cups.

Pour the water into a clean pan, add 1¼ cups of the sugar, the cloves, and cinnamon stick, and heat gently, stirring, until the sugar has dissolved. Raise the heat and bring the mixture to a boil, then stir in the peels. Remove the pan from the heat and allow contents to cool, then transfer to an air-tight container and leave in a cool place for 2 days.

Drain the syrup into a clean pan, add the remaining sugar, and stir over low heat until the sugar has dissolved. Add the peels and simmer for 1–1½ hours or until transparent. Pour the contents of the pan into a nonmetallic bowl, cover, and leave in a cool place for 2–3 weeks.

*O*RANGES

Drain off the syrup and transfer the peels to a wire rack placed over a tray. Put in a warm place or in the oven no hotter than 125°F and leave for several hours until the peels are dry and no longer feel sticky.

Carefully pack the peels into containers, laying waxed paper or parchment between each layer. Store in a cool, dark, dry place for up to 1 year.

Variation: To make plain candied peel, simply omit the spices and follow the method above.

Orange Curd with Candied Orange Peel

Tangy pieces of homemade candied peel, either spiced or plain, make an interesting texture change in this smooth, buttery curd. If you do not have time to make the Candied Orange Peel, you can use store-bought candied peel.

MAKES ABOUT 2 CUPS

grated zest and juice of 4 large oranges
1 cup Candied Orange Peel (see page 66),
  chopped
1 cup unsalted butter, diced
scant 1 cup superfine sugar
6 large egg yolks

Put the orange zest and juice, candied orange peel, butter, and sugar in a heatproof bowl or double boiler and place over a saucepan of gently simmering water; do not allow the bottom of the bowl to sit in the water. Heat the mixture gently, stirring constantly, until all the sugar has dissolved and the butter has melted.

Strain the egg yolks into the bowl and continue to stir the mixture over gently simmering water until the curd thickens. This should take 30–40 minutes. Stir the mixture occasionally at first, more frequently as the cooking progresses, and constantly toward the end of the cooking so that the curd cooks evenly and does not curdle. The water must not boil.

Pour the curd into warm, clean, dry jars. Cover, seal, and process (see pages 12–13). Store in a cool, dark, dry place or in the refrigerator. The curd must be refrigerated after opening.

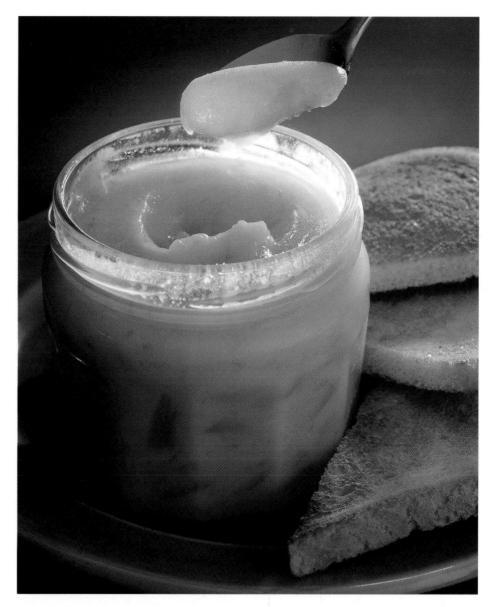

Above: Orange Curd with Candied Orange Peel makes a delicious buttery spread that is the ideal partner for toasted white bread.

Honeyed Peel

This is somewhat easier and quicker to make than candied peel (see page 66).

MAKES ABOUT 2½ CUPS

peel of 4 small thin-skinned oranges
1⅓ cups clear honey

Scrape all the white pith off the peel, then cut the peel into strips. Blanch the peel strips in boiling water for 5 minutes. Drain and rinse under running cold water, then dry thoroughly on paper towels.

Make a layer of peel in a clean, dry jar and pour in 1 tablespoon honey. Repeat the layering until all the peel and honey have been used.

Close the jar tightly and store in a cool, dark, dry place for 3 months, shaking the jar occasionally and topping up with more honey if necessary so that the peel remains completely covered.

Serving Suggestion
Wherever you would use candied peel in desserts, cakes, and cookies, in rice pudding and ice cream; mix with dried fruit as a stuffing for baked apples; add to apple or pear pies or tarts.

Orange Peel Scrolls

The luxurious taste of this sweet-tangy preserve belies its simplicity. It makes use of the peel, an ingredient that is more usually thrown away and wasted.

peel of 6 thin-skinned oranges, cut into strips
1¼ cups sugar
1 teaspoon lemon juice

Place the peel in a large saucepan with a generous 1 cup water, and simmer for 40 minutes or until it is soft. Drain well,

reserving the water. When cool enough to handle, roll up each strip of orange peel and thread it onto a length of thread knotted at one end, pushing the scrolls together so that they do not unroll (see below). When all the scrolls are in place, knot the thread again. Add the sugar and lemon juice to the water and heat gently in the pan, stirring, until the sugar has dissolved. Raise the heat and bring the mixture to a boil, then add the string of orange peel and simmer for 1 hour or until the syrup has been thoroughly absorbed into the peel, and the peel is translucent.

Remove the string of peel, cut one knot, then, using a fork, push the scrolls from the thread into a warm, clean, dry jar. If necessary, boil the syrup vigorously until it is thick enough to coat the back of a spoon (keep the jar warm in a low oven or on the stove while doing this). Pour the syrup into the jar to cover the scrolls completely. Cover and keep for 1–2 days before eating. Store in a cool, dark, dry place for 6–12 months.

Serving Suggestion
Serve the scrolls and some of the syrup with whipped cream or thick yogurt and plain lady fingers or crisp cookies; serve with creamy or chocolate desserts; roll in granulated sugar and serve with coffee.

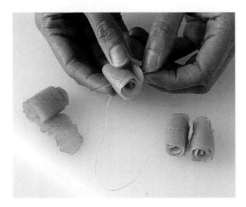

Making Orange Peel Scrolls: Use a needle to string the scrolls onto a thread. Knot both ends of the thread to prevent them from unrolling.

Orange Shrub

A shrub is an old-fashioned sweetened alcoholic drink. Unless you have some really fruity-tasting oranges, use freshly squeezed orange juice. Citric acid freshens and lifts the flavor.

MAKES ABOUT 3 CUPS

2 strips of orange zest, chopped
½ cup freshly squeezed orange juice, slightly warmed
⅓ cup superfine sugar
about 1 teaspoon citric acid (optional)
2½ cups white or dark rum or brandy

Put the orange zest in a small saucepan of boiling water. Return the water to a boil for 1 minute, then drain.

Put the orange zest and juice, sugar, and citric acid, if using, in a clean, dry bottle and shake to dissolve the sugar. Add the rum or brandy and shake again, then cover and leave in a cool, dark, dry place for 2 weeks or until clear, shaking the bottle daily.

Strain through a double thickness of cheesecloth and pour into a clean, dry bottle. Close the bottle (see pages 12–13) and store in a cool, dark, dry place for 2 months before drinking.

Vin d'Orange

This aperitif comes from southern France where it is sipped leisurely at many a café.

MAKES 5 CUPS

2 large oranges
1 cup plus 2 tablespoons superfine sugar
1 quart dry white wine
½ cup Armagnac

Pare the zest from the oranges, taking care not to include any white pith. Put the zest in a bottle, add the remaining ingredients, and close the bottle.

TANGERINES

Shake the bottle, then leave it in a sunny or warm place for about 2 weeks, shaking the bottle daily.

Strain the wine through a nonmetallic funnel lined with cheesecloth into a clean, dry bottle. Close the bottle (see pages 12–13). The wine is now ready for drinking.

Tangerine Ratafia

A ratafia is a fruit liqueur made by steeping fruit in alcohol for a couple of months to produce a deliciously scented sweet drink; the sweetness can be altered by adjusting the amount of sugar.

MAKES ABOUT 2½ CUPS

6 tangerines
½ teaspoon coriander seeds, lightly crushed
3-inch piece cinnamon stick, broken into 3 pieces
2 cups vodka, gin, or brandy
about 1 cup superfine sugar

Halve the tangerines, squeeze the juice from the fruit, then pour it into a clean, dry jar. Pull the flesh and membranes away from the fruit peel and discard them. Cut the peel into thin strips and add to the jar with the coriander seeds, cinnamon pieces, liquor, and sugar to taste.

Cover and seal the jar and shake the ingredients together. Store in a cool, dark, dry place for 2 months, shaking the jar occasionally.

Strain the ratafia through a nonmetallic funnel lined with cheesecloth into a clean, dry bottle. Close the bottle (see pages 12–13). The ratafia is now ready to drink.

Variation: *Satsuma or Clementine Ratafia* Substitute satsumas or clementines for the tangerines.

Right: Vin d'Orange and Tangerine Ratafia are ideal for drinking on a hot summer's day.

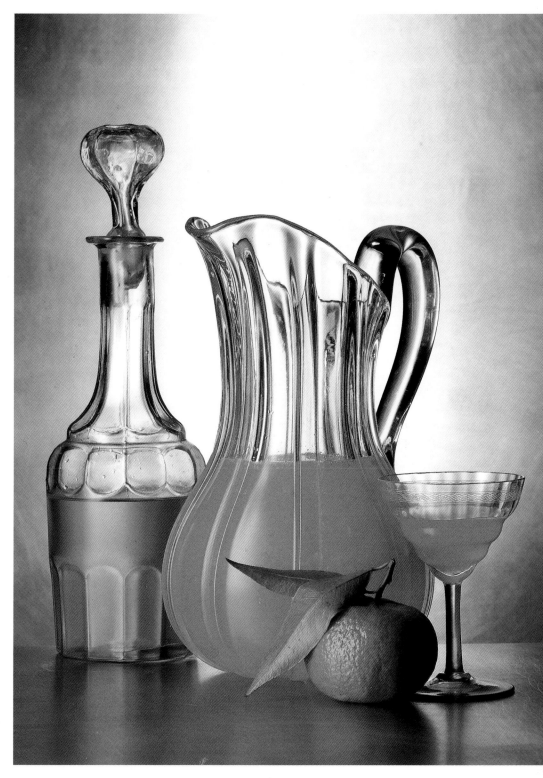

Tangerine and Apple Jam

MAKES ABOUT 3⅔ CUPS

1¼ pounds tangerines
12 ounces cooking apples
4 cups warmed sugar (see page 7)
juice of 2 lemons

Halve and chop the tangerines, including the peel, removing and reserving the seeds.

Peel, core, and slice the apples. Tie the apple cores and peel and the tangerine seeds in a cheesecloth bag. Put all the fruit, peel, and 2½ cups water in a large saucepan, tie the loose end of the cheesecloth bag string on the pan handle so that the bag is suspended in the mixture, and bring to a boil, then cover and simmer for 1 hour.

Scoop out the cheesecloth bag with a slotted spoon and press the bag firmly with the back of a metal spoon so that the juices run back into the pan.

Over low heat, stir in the sugar until it has dissolved. Add the lemon juice, then boil for about 20 minutes, stirring, until setting point is reached (see page 17).

Remove the pan from the heat and skim the scum from the surface with a slotted spoon. Ladle the jam into warm, clean, dry jars. Cover, seal, and process (see pages 12–13). Leave overnight to set slightly. Store in a cool, dark, dry place.

Serving Suggestion
Use in apple fritters; added to rhubarb for a crumble, pie, or cobbler; spread beneath apple slices in an apple pie; as a filling for warm scones or a roulade.

Tangerine Curd

For extra spice, you can add a little grated fresh ginger or a few lightly crushed cardamom seeds.

MAKES ABOUT 2 CUPS

finely grated zest and juice from 1 pound tangerines
finely grated zest and juice of 1 lemon
½ cup unsalted butter
1⅓ cups superfine sugar
4 large eggs, lightly beaten

Put the tangerine and lemon zests and juice, the butter, and sugar in a heatproof bowl or double boiler and place over a saucepan of gently simmering water; do not allow the bottom of the bowl to sit in the water. Heat gently, stirring constantly, until the sugar has dissolved and the butter has melted.

Strain in the eggs and continue to stir over gently simmering water for 30–40 minutes or until the curd thickens enough to coat the back of the spoon. Stir occasionally at first, then more frequently as the cooking progresses, and constantly toward the end so that the curd cooks evenly and does not curdle. The water must not boil.

Pour the curd into warm, clean, dry jars. Cover, seal, and process (see pages 12–13). Store in a cool, dark, dry place or the refrigerator. Refrigerate after opening.

Tangerine Marmalade

Tangerines make a very well-flavored, clear, fruity marmalade.

MAKES ABOUT 2 QUARTS

2 pounds tangerines
juice of 2 large lemons
7 cups warmed sugar (see page 7)

Cut the tangerines in half and squeeze out the juice. Scrape the membranes from the tangerines and tie in a cheesecloth bag with the seeds. Cut the peel into thin strips.

Put the tangerine and lemon juices and the peel into a large saucepan with 7½ cups water. Tie the loose end of the cheesecloth bag string onto the pan handle so that the bag is suspended in the mixture. Bring to a boil, then simmer for about 1½ hours or until the peel is tender and the pan contents have reduced by half.

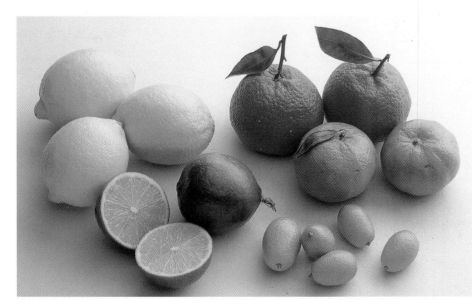

Left, clockwise from front right: Kumquats, limes, lemons, clementines, and satsumas.

Scoop out the cheesecloth bag with a slotted spoon and press the bag firmly with the back of a metal spoon so that the juices flow back into the pan. Discard the bag.

Over low heat, add the warmed sugar and stir until dissolved. Raise the heat and boil vigorously for about 15 minutes, stirring if necessary, until setting point is reached (see page 17). Remove from the heat. Skim the scum from the surface with a slotted spoon. Leave to stand for 10–15 minutes, then stir and ladle into warm, clean, dry jars. Cover, seal, and process (see pages 12–13). Leave overnight. Store in a cool, dark, dry place.

Serving Suggestion
Serve with croissants for breakfast; use to sandwich the layers of sponge cakes.

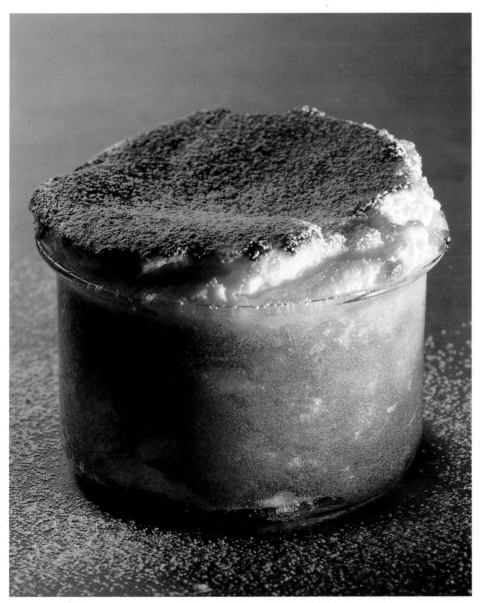

Tangerine Marmalade Soufflés

Tangerine Marmalade turns inexpensive ingredients into a very special dinner-party dessert.

SERVES 4

2 large eggs, separated
1 large egg yolk
⅓ cup sugar
1½ tablespoons all-purpose flour, sifted
1 cup milk
2 tablespoons Tangerine Marmalade (see page 70)
2 tablespoons whiskey (optional)

Preheat the oven to 400°F. Lightly butter four 1-cup ramekins.

Whisk together all the egg yolks and the sugar until thick and pale. Gently fold in the sifted flour with a metal spoon.

Bring the milk to a boil in a heavy saucepan, then slowly pour it into the egg yolk mixture, stirring. Return the mixture to the rinsed saucepan and heat gently, stirring, until thickened; do not allow it to boil. Remove from the heat and stir in the marmalade and whiskey if using.

Whisk the egg whites until stiff but not dry. Stir 2 tablespoons into the marmalade mixture to lighten it, then carefully fold in the remainder. Divide between the ramekins. Bake in the center of the oven for about 13 minutes or until well risen and lightly set. Serve immediately.

Left: Light, fruity, and irresistible, Tangerine Marmalade Soufflés make the perfect ending to a special dinner.

Grapefruit and Apple Curd

MAKES 3–4⅓ CUPS

**2 pounds cooking apples, peeled, cored,
   and sliced
1 cup unsalted butter, diced
2 cups superfine sugar
4 large eggs, lightly beaten
grated zest and juice of 1 large grapefruit**

Place the apples in a large saucepan with a small amount of water, cover the pan, and cook gently until the apples are soft and pulpy. Transfer the apples to a heatproof bowl or double boiler, place over a saucepan of simmering water and add the butter and sugar. Do not allow the bottom of the bowl to sit in the water. Heat the mixture gently, stirring constantly, until all the sugar has dissolved and the butter has melted.

Strain in the eggs, add the grapefruit zest and juice, and continue to stir over gently simmering water until the curd thickens enough to coat the back of the spoon, which can take 30–40 minutes. Stir occasionally at first, more frequently as the cooking progresses, and constantly toward the end so that the curd cooks evenly and does not curdle. The water must not boil.

Pour the curd into warm, clean, dry jars. Cover, seal, and process (see pages 12–13). Store in a cool, dark, dry place or the refrigerator. Refrigerate after opening.

Pink Grapefruit Marmalade

MAKES ABOUT 6⅔ CUPS

**2 pink grapefruit
2 lemons
9 cups warmed sugar (see page 7)**

Cut the grapefruit and lemons in half and squeeze out the juice. Reserve the seeds and any membrane that has come away during squeezing and place on a square of cheesecloth. Roughly chop the lemon halves, add to the cheesecloth, and then tie into a bag.

Quarter each grapefruit half, then cut across into strips. Put the strips, grapefruit and lemon juices, and 9 cups water into a large saucepan and tie the loose end of string of the cheesecloth bag onto the pan handle so that the bag is suspended in the mixture. Bring the mixture to a boil, then simmer for about 45 minutes or until the peel is soft.

Remove the cheesecloth bag with a slotted spoon and press it firmly with the back of a metal spoon so that the juices run back into the pan. Discard the bag.

Over low heat, stir in the warmed sugar until it has dissolved, then raise the heat and boil vigorously for 10–15 minutes, stirring as necessary, until setting point is reached (see page 17).

Remove from the heat and skim the scum from the surface with a slotted spoon. Leave to stand for 10–15 minutes, then stir and ladle into warm, clean, dry jars. Cover, seal, and process (see pages 12–13). Leave overnight to set. Store in a cool, dark, dry place.

Kumquats in Vodka and Cointreau

Kumquats are the smallest of the citrus fruits and have a bittersweet flavor.

MAKES 4 CUPS

**¾ cup plus 2 tablespoons sugar
2¼ pounds kumquats
1¼ cups vodka
⅔ cup Cointreau**

Mix the sugar and 2½ cups water in a large saucepan and heat gently, stirring, until the sugar dissolves. Meanwhile, prick the kumquats all over with a large embroidery needle. Add them to the pan and simmer for about 15 minutes or until the skins feel soft; pierce with a fine skewer to test.

Using a slotted spoon, remove the kumquats from the syrup and pack into warm, clean, dry jars. Pour the vodka and Cointreau over the kumquats, then fill to the top with the reserved syrup.

Cover and seal the jars (see pages 12–13). Invert them gently to mix the liquids. Store in a cool, dark, dry place for at least 1 month before eating.

Serving Suggestion
Serve with thick yogurt, creamy rice pudding, or slices of gingerbread.

Pickled Kumquats with Cardamom

Kumquats are unlike other citrus fruits in that the peel is sweeter than the flesh. Their tart-sweetness works well with honey and spices.

MAKES 2 CUPS

**18 ounces kumquats
1 teaspoon sea salt
¾ cup plus 2 tablespoons white wine vinegar
¼ cup clear honey
3 cardamom pods, crushed
1 whole clove
½-inch piece of fresh ginger,
   thinly sliced, then cut into fine shreds**

Cut the kumquats in half, then put them in a large saucepan with the salt and add water to cover. Bring to a boil, then simmer for 5 minutes. Drain the kumquats, discarding any seeds.

𝒦UMQUATS

Put the vinegar, honey, cardamom pods, clove, and ginger into a pan and heat gently, stirring, until the honey has dissolved. Raise the heat and bring the mixture to a boil, then add the kumquats.

Ladle the kumquats and the liquid into warm, clean, dry jars. Cover with acid-proof lids, seal, and process (see pages 12–13). Store in a cool, dark, dry place for 1 month before eating.

Serving Suggestion

Add a generous spoonful to the cooking juices of roast duck or pork; serve with duck or game terrines.

Kumquat Conserve

This is fruity, sharp, and sweet, with a little kick of whiskey.

MAKES ABOUT 4 CUPS

1½ pounds ripe kumquats
3⅓ cups sugar
¼ cup whiskey

Using a sharp knife, chop the kumquats into coarse chunks and then layer them with the sugar in a bowl. Cover and leave in a cool place for 1 day.

Transfer the contents of the bowl to a large saucepan, add 1¼ cups water, and heat gently, stirring, until the sugar has dissolved. Raise the heat and boil vigorously for 10 minutes or until the liquid is syrupy.

Remove from the heat, stir in the whiskey, and leave to stand for 10–15 minutes. Stir, then ladle into warm, clean, dry jars. Cover, seal, and process (see pages 12–13). Leave overnight to set. Store the conserve in a cool, dark, dry place.

Right: Lime Shred Marmalade and Kumquat Conserve make a deliciously tangy addition to the breakfast table.

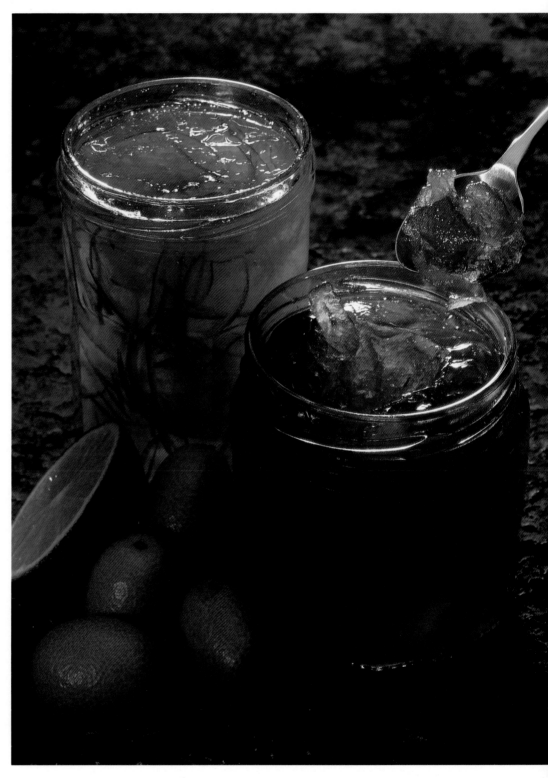

Chicken Tagine with Preserved Lemons and Olives

In this Moroccan dish, the mellow flavor of the preserved lemons is beautifully complemented by pinky-brown Moroccan olives; if you cannot find them, substitute Greek Kalamata olives. Preserved lemons make this dish extra special, but you can substitute a fresh lemon, if desired.

SERVES 4

1 Spanish onion, finely chopped
2–3 tablespoons olive oil
3 garlic cloves, chopped
salt and freshly ground black pepper
¾ teaspoon ground ginger
1 teaspoon ground cinnamon
½ teaspoon saffron threads, toasted
**   and crushed**
1 chicken, about 3½ pounds
3 cups chicken stock or water
4 ounces pinky-brown Moroccan olives, rinsed
1 Moroccan Preserved Lemon (see page 75),
**   flesh discarded if desired, rinsed and chopped**
large bunch of fresh cilantro, finely chopped
large bunch of fresh parsley, finely chopped

Gently sauté the onion in the oil, stirring frequently, until it is soft and golden.

Meanwhile, crush the garlic with a pinch of salt, then work in the ginger, cinnamon, saffron, and a little pepper. Stir into the onions and continue cooking until fragrant.

Put the chicken in a heavy saucepan or flameproof casserole that it just fits, spread the onion mixture all over, then add the stock or water and bring to simmering. Cover and simmer very gently for about 1¼ hours, turning the chicken over 2 or 3 times.

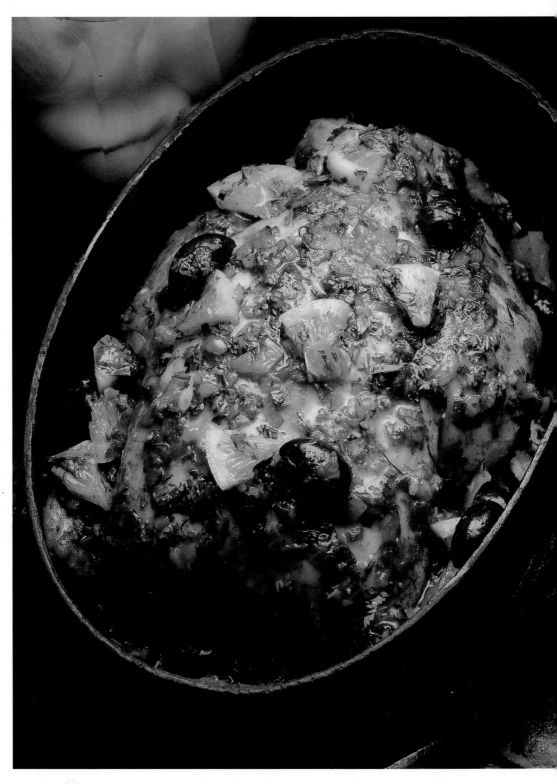

Right: Chicken Tagine with Preserved Lemons and Olives makes an exotic dinner dish.

Add the olives, preserved lemon, cilantro, and parsley, cover again, and cook for another 15 minutes or until the chicken is very tender.

Taste the sauce – if the flavor needs to be more concentrated, transfer the chicken to a warm, shallow serving dish, cover, and keep warm, then boil the cooking juices to reduce them to a rich sauce. Tilt the pan and skim off the surplus fat if desired, then pour the sauce over the chicken.

Moroccan Preserved Lemons

Lemons lose their sharpness when preserved in salt. The unique flavor and silken texture that develops when you use this technique is a characteristic of North African, especially Moroccan, cooking. Yet the lemons also make a novel addition to non-Moroccan dishes. You will find that these lemons are easy to prepare and thin-skinned lemons yield the most juice. Traditionally, only the peel of the preserved fruit is used, but I usually include the flesh as well.

Once the jar has been opened, the fruit will keep for up to 1 year unrefrigerated (do not worry if a lacy white film appears on top of the jar or on the lemons, as it is quite harmless – simply rinse it off); a layer of olive oil floated on the surface will help to preserve freshness.

7 tablespoons sea salt
7 plump, juicy lemons, preferably thin-skinned

Put 1 teaspoon coarse salt in the bottom of a clean, dry jar. Holding a lemon over a plate to catch the juice, cut lengthwise 4 times as if about to quarter it, but do not cut quite through – leave the pieces joined. Ease out any seeds. Pack 1 tablespoon salt into the cuts, then close them up around the salt

and put the lemon in the jar. Repeat with 5 more fruit, packing them tightly and pressing each layer down to expel any air before adding the next layer, until the jar is full.

Squeeze another lemon and pour the juice over the fruit. Sprinkle with more coarse salt and pour in boiling water to cover the fruit. Close the jar tightly and keep in a warm place for 3–4 weeks before using.

Serving Suggestion
Add to spicy lamb, chicken, and fish casseroles; use the juice in salad dressings.

Lemon and Passionfruit Curd

This delectable spread combines the sharp, clean taste of lemon with scented passionfruit.

MAKES ABOUT 1⅓ CUPS

1 teaspoon finely grated lemon zest
½ cup lemon juice (about 2½ lemons)
6 tablespoons unsalted butter, diced
generous 1 cup superfine sugar
3 large eggs, lightly beaten
2 passionfruit, halved and pulp scooped out

Put the lemon zest and juice, butter, and sugar in a heatproof bowl or double boiler and place over a saucepan of gently simmering water; do not allow the base of the bowl to sit in the water. Heat gently, stirring constantly, until the sugar has dissolved and the butter melted.

Strain in the eggs and continue to stir over gently simmering water until the curd thickens enough to coat the back of the spoon, which can take 30–40 minutes. Stir occasionally at first, more frequently as the cooking progresses, and constantly toward the end so that the curd cooks evenly and does not curdle. The water must not boil.

Remove the bowl from the heat and stir in the passionfruit pulp. Pour the curd into warm, clean, dry jars. Cover, seal, and process (see pages 12–13). Store in a cool, dark, dry place or the refrigerator. Refrigerate after opening.

Serving Suggestion
Diluted with extra lemon juice and some rum, white or dark, this makes a superb sauce for spooning over a cheesecake.

St. Clement's Cordial

Mixtures of orange and lemon are often called St. Clement's after the English nursery rhyme, "The Bells of St. Clement's." If you prefer a smooth drink, strain the cordial through a nonmetallic sieve lined with a double thickness of cheesecloth; squeeze the pulp in the cheesecloth in order to extract the maximum amount of juice.

MAKES ABOUT 6 CUPS

about 6 large juicy oranges
about 3 lemons
3⅓ cups sugar

Grate the zest from 1½ oranges and 1½ lemons. Squeeze the juice from all the oranges to make about 2¼ cups juice and from all the lemons to make about 1 cup.

Put the fruit juices and zests into a large saucepan, add the sugar, and heat gently, stirring, until the sugar has dissolved. Raise the heat slightly and bring to just below the boiling point.

Immediately remove the pan from the heat and pour the cordial into warm, clean, dry bottles. Cover and process in a water bath (see page 13). Alternatively, leave the cordial to cool, then pour it into cold bottles and keep in the refrigerator for up to 1 month.

Lime Curd

Use limes in place of lemons to make a fruity, tangy change to the more traditional lemon curd (for lemon curd recipe, see variation below).

MAKES ABOUT 2 CUPS

finely grated zest and juice of 5 large
 juicy limes
½ cup unsalted butter, diced
1½ cups superfine sugar
4 large eggs, lightly beaten

Put the lime zest and juice, butter, and sugar in a heatproof bowl or double boiler and place over a saucepan of gently simmering water; do not allow the bottom of the bowl to sit in the water. Heat the mixture gently, stirring constantly, until all the sugar has dissolved and the butter has melted.

Strain the eggs into the bowl and continue to stir over gently simmering water until the curd thickens enough to coat the back of the spoon. This should take about 30–40 minutes. Stir occasionally at first, more frequently as the cooking progresses, then constantly toward the end of the cooking time so that the curd cooks evenly and does not curdle. Do not allow the water to boil.

Pour the curd into warm, clean, dry jars. Cover, seal, and process (see pages 12–13). Store in a cool dark, dry place or the refrigerator. Refrigerate after opening.

Variation: *Lemon Curd*
Use 4 medium plump lemons in place of the limes. Follow the recipe above. Makes about 2 cups.

Lime Shred Marmalade

My grandmother had a particular passion for Lime Shred Marmalade. She would spread it very thickly on her breakfast toast (white bread had to be bought specially – this marmalade goes better with white bread than brown). I used to make her a batch for Christmas. One year, as a special treat, I used the peel from Thai kaffir limes. The marmalade was eaten with even greater relish, so from then on I always used kaffir lime peel (the rest of the fruit is never used).

MAKES ABOUT 6⅔ CUPS

1½ pounds limes (about 12) *or* 1½ pounds limes
 (for flesh only) and 1 pound kaffir limes (for
 peel only)
7 cups warmed sugar (see page 7)

Peel the limes thinly, then cut the peel into thin strips. Thinly slice the flesh, reserving any juice, and tie the seeds into a cheesecloth bag.

Put the fruit, any reserved juice, the peel, and 7 cups water into a large saucepan and tie the loose end of string onto the pan handle so that the bag is suspended in the mixture. Simmer for about 1 hour or until the peel is tender and the contents of the pan reduced by about half.

Scoop out the cheesecloth bag with a slotted spoon and, wearing rubber gloves to protect your hands from the hot liquid, squeeze firmly to press the juices back into the pan. Discard the cheesecloth bag.

Over low heat, stir in the warmed sugar until it has dissolved. Raise the heat and boil vigorously for 10–15 minutes, stirring as necessary, until setting point is reached (see page 17).

Remove from the heat and skim off any scum from the surface with a slotted spoon. Leave to stand for 10–15 minutes, then stir and ladle into warm, clean, dry jars. Cover, seal, and process (see pages 12–13). Leave overnight. Store in a cool, dark, dry place.

Variation: *Lemon Shred Marmalade*
Substitute the same weight of lemons for the limes and follow the method above. Makes about 6⅔ cups.

Lime Chutney

If you can resist dipping into this pungent chutney (and I'll bet you can't), it is best to keep it for up to 1 year before eating to allow the flavors to develop fully. This chutney is the perfect accompaniment to all manner of spicy foods.

MAKES ABOUT 6⅔ CUPS

2 pounds large limes, thinly sliced
1 pound onions, finely chopped
¼ cup sea salt
1 tablespoon coriander seeds
2 tablespoons plus 1 teaspoon allspice berries
1 tablespoon plus 1 teaspoon whole cardamom
 pods, crushed
4 dried red chilies, seeded if desired and
 chopped
2 ounces fresh ginger, peeled and grated
2½ cups white wine vinegar
2¼ cups warmed superfine sugar (see page 7)

Put the limes, onions, and salt in a large nonmetallic bowl. Place the coriander seeds, allspice berries, and cardamom pods on a square of cheesecloth and tie together with string to make a bag. Stir the bag into the bowl. Cover the bowl and leave in a cool place for 1 day.

Transfer the contents of the bowl to a large saucepan and stir in the chilies, ginger, and vinegar. Bring the mixture to a boil, then lower the heat and simmer for 1½ hours, stirring occasionally.

Add the warmed sugar to the saucepan and stir until all the sugar has dissolved. Raise the heat and bring to a boil, then lower the heat and simmer, stirring occasionally, until the chutney is thick and there is no free liquid. Scoop out the cheesecloth bag and discard. Ladle the chutney into warm, clean, dry jars, taking care not to trap any air bubbles. Cover with acid-proof lids, seal, and process (see pages 12–13). Store the chutney in a cool, dark, dry place for at least 1 month or up to 1 year before eating.

Serving Suggestion
Serve this chutney with curries and other spicy dishes.

Indian Sweet-Sour Lime Pickle

Long pickling causes lime wedges to turn almost gelatinous and gives them a wonderful flavor.

MAKES ABOUT 3½ CUPS

12–14 limes
3-inch piece of fresh ginger, peeled, thinly sliced, and then cut into fine strips
4 garlic cloves, quartered lengthwise (optional)
6 teaspoons sea salt
about 3 fresh green chilies
1 cup white wine vinegar
2 cups sugar

Cut 6 limes lengthwise into 6 wedges each. Put a layer of lime wedges in the bottom of a wide-necked jar, with their cut sides facing outward. Sprinkle with some of the ginger and some of the garlic if using and about 1 teaspoon of the salt. Repeat the layering process, pressing down on the ingredients slightly to expel air and adding a chilli here and there, until the jar is filled to within ½–¾ inch from the top.

Squeeze the juice from the remaining limes to make a scant 1 cup. Pour into a saucepan with the vinegar and sugar and heat gently, stirring, until the sugar has dissolved, then simmer gently until the mixture becomes slightly syrupy.

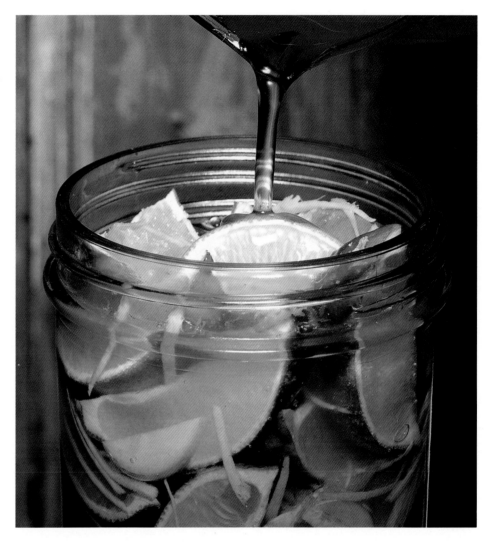

Pour the mixture into the jar and rotate the jar to expel any air bubbles. If the top layer of limes floats to the surface, weight them down with some waxed paper. Cover the jar with an acid-proof lid, seal, and process (see pages 12–13).

Leave in a sunny or warm place for 1 month, then store for another 2–4 weeks at room temperature before eating.

Serving Suggestions
Serve with spicy grilled chicken, Indian spinach dishes, or to accompany salmon; use as a filling in cheese sandwiches.

Above: Indian Sweet-Sour Lime Pickle makes an attractive and zesty accompaniment to a wide variety of spicy dishes.

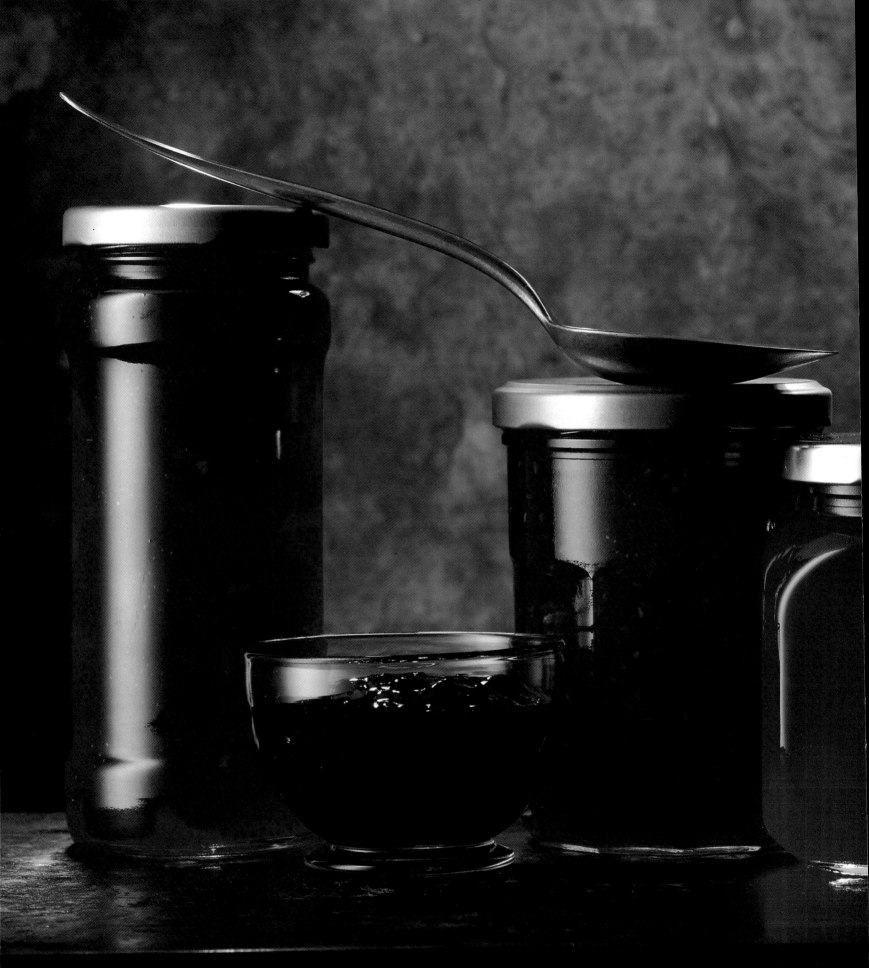

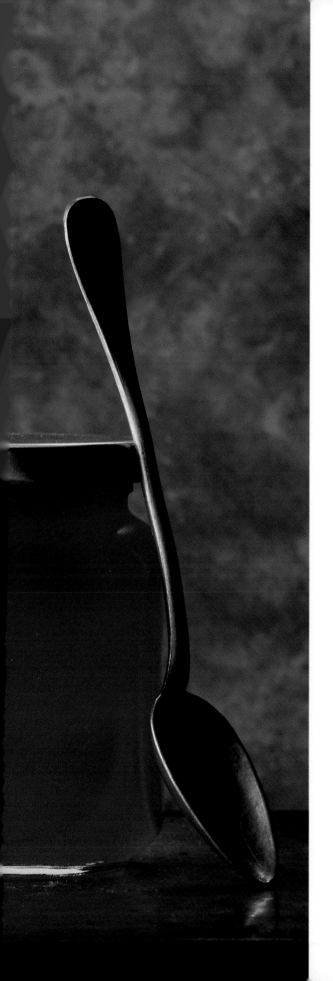

SOFT FRUITS

Soft fruits have always been prime candidates for preserving because they traditionally have limited growing seasons. However, by using genetics and selection, growers have extended natural seasons, but the quantities are small, the prices high, and the flavors disappointing. (Flavor is not just a question of exposure to the sun but also of comparatively slow ripening.) As far as I am concerned, soft fruits still remain a seasonal crop. Some of the most popular, as well as the most innovative, of preserves can be made from soft fruit. In this chapter you will find preserves varying from traditional Blackberry Jam (see page 80) to Spiced Cranberry and Apple Sauce (see page 85) and Red Summer Fruits Preserve (see page 91). When preparing soft fruits for cooking, handle them gently and, unless they are very dirty, do not rinse them in water. If they are slightly dirty, wipe them carefully with a damp cloth; otherwise, it is best to keep them dry.

Left, from left to right: Strawberry Conserve, Blackberry Jam, Red Summer Fruits Preserve, and Superlative Red Currant Jelly.

Blackberry Conserve

blackberries
sugar
lemon juice

Preheat the oven to the lowest setting.

Weigh the berries and reserve some for topping up the jars later.

Pack the remaining blackberries firmly into clean, dry jars (use 500ml/2¼ cup jars, if you have them), sprinkling in about 1 tablespoon lemon juice and 7 tablespoons sugar for every 1 pound fruit. Put the reserved berries in a separate jar.

Put all the jars of fruit on the bottom shelf of the oven for 45–50 minutes or until the jars are thoroughly hot. The fruit will have shrunk a little, so top up the jar with the reserved berries. Pour boiling water into the jars to cover the fruit completely and seal immediately. Leave overnight before eating. Store in a cool, dark, dry place.

Serving Suggestion

Serve over ice cream or plain sponge cake and accompany with whipped cream; serve with muffins or scones.

Blackberry Jam

Recipes always used to specify using unripe blackberries to get a good set, but now, with commercial liquid pectin so readily available, this is not vital. The length of time you will need to cook the fruit, if, indeed, you need to cook it at all, will depend on the blackberries; reduce the water in relation to the reduction in the cooking time.

MAKES ABOUT 4⅔ CUPS

2¼ pounds blackberries
juice of ½ lemon
commercial liquid pectin or ⅓ cup pectin
  extract (see page 7)

5 cups warmed sugar (see page 7)
2 tablespoons gin (optional)

Put the blackberries, lemon juice, and ¼ cup water in a large saucepan, cover, and heat very gently, shaking the pan occasionally, for 10–15 minutes or until the fruit is soft.

Carefully stir in the pectin extract and the sugar over low heat, taking care not to break up the berries, until they are dissolved (if using commercial pectin, follow the manufacturer's directions). Raise the heat and boil vigorously for about 4 minutes or until setting point is reached (see page 17).

Remove from the heat and stir in the gin if using. Ladle into warm, clean, dry jars. Cover, seal, and process (see pages 12–13). Leave overnight. Store the jam in a cool, dark, dry place.

Variation: *Raspberry Jam*
Use 2 pounds raspberries, commercial liquid pectin or 2⅓ cups pectin extract (see page 7), and the juice of 1 lemon. Gently heat all the ingredients, stirring carefully, until the sugar has dissolved. Proceed with the recipe above. Makes about 5⅓ cups.

Blackberry Spread

According to an old English saying, you should pick blackberries before the end of September, when the devil spits on them. If he does, he didn't spoil the wonderful dark color or rich flavor of the blackberry spread I made last year.

MAKES ABOUT 4 CUPS

3 pounds blackberries
1 tablespoon lemon juice
warmed sugar (see page 7)

Put the blackberries and lemon juice in a large saucepan, add barely enough water to cover, and bring to a boil, then simmer for about 15 minutes or until the fruit is soft and pulpy.

Press the fruit through a nonmetallic sieve. Measure the purée and return it to the rinsed pan. Add 1¾ cups sugar for every 2½ cups purée and heat gently, stirring, until the sugar has dissolved. Raise the heat and boil gently, stirring frequently, for 45–55 minutes or until the mixture is so thick that when the spoon is drawn across the bottom of the pan, a clear trail is left.

Spoon into warm, clean, dry jars or into lightly oiled decorative molds; do not trap any air bubbles. Cover, seal, and process (see pages 12–13). Store in a cool, dark, dry place for 2–3 months before eating.

Serving Suggestion

This is an excellent accompaniment to mature Cheddar cheese, crusty, firm-textured white bread, and unsalted butter.

Blackberry Cordial

This is an old-fashioned sharp, sweet cordial. Blackberries should be large, ripe, and glossy, so pass over any small, hard, seedy fruit – they really aren't worth bothering with.

MAKES ABOUT 2 QUARTS

2 pounds blackberries
2½ cups white wine vinegar
2¼ cups sugar
⅔ cup clear honey

Put the fruit and vinegar in a nonmetallic bowl. Crush the fruit with a wooden spoon, then cover the bowl and leave in a cool place for 1 week, stirring and pressing the fruit 2 or 3 times a day.

Strain the contents of the bowl through a nonmetallic sieve into a pan, pressing firmly on the sieve with the wooden spoon to extract as much juice as possible. Stir in the sugar and honey and heat gently until the sugar has dissolved. Raise the heat and boil for 5 minutes, stirring as necessary.

$\mathscr{B}$LACKBERRIES

Pour the cordial into warm, clean, dry bottles and leave to cool, then cover, seal, and process (see pages 12–13). Store in a cool, dark, dry place.

Serving Suggestion
Add 1 tablespoonful to a mug of hot water as a soothing cough and cold reliever or as a pleasant drink at bedtime or on a cold day.

Below: A combination of wild fruits produces this delicious Blackberry and Elderberry Jelly.

Blackberry and Elderberry Jelly

Long but gentle cooking produces this fruity-flavored jelly.

MAKES 3½ CUPS

3 large lemons
6 pounds blackberries and elderberries
warmed sugar (see page 7)

Squeeze the juice from the lemons and reserve the seeds. Put the juice, seeds, berries and 6 tablespoons water in a heavy casserole and stir together. Lay waxed paper on the fruit, then cover the casserole.

Cook in a very low oven for a few hours or until the fruit is very tender.

Crush the fruit with a potato masher, then pour the contents of the casserole into a scalded jelly bag suspended over a nonmetallic bowl and leave to strain, undisturbed, in a cool place for 8–12 hours.

Measure the juice and put into a pan with 2¼ cups sugar for every 2½ cups juice. Heat gently, stirring, until the sugar has dissolved, then raise the heat and boil vigorously for about 15 minutes or until setting point is reached (see page 17). Immediately ladle into warm, clean, dry jars. Cover, seal, and process (see pages 12–13). Leave overnight to set. Store in a cool, dark, dry place.

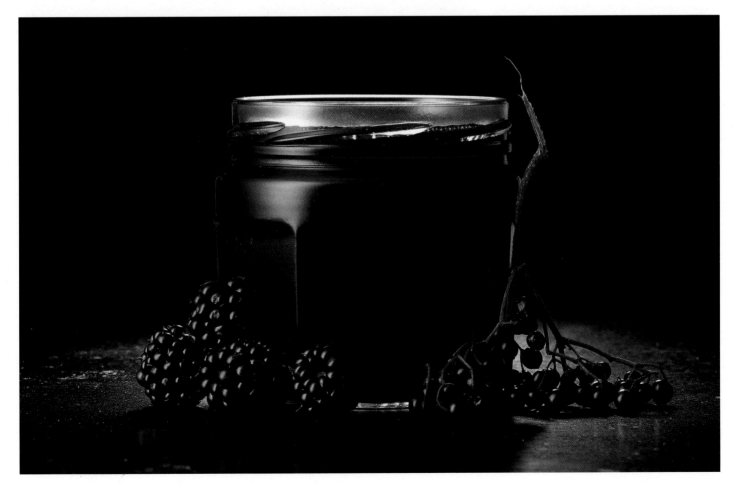

Quick Savory Blackberry Jelly

Simple straining through an ordinary nonmetallic sieve, instead of lengthy straining through a jelly bag, is all that is needed to produce this magnificent dark, firm, richly flavored jelly. If serving it as an accompaniment, present it on a white plate or in a white bowl to show off its deep color.

MAKES ABOUT 4 CUPS

1 tablespoon whole cloves
2 cinnamon sticks
1 teaspoon allspice berries
4 pounds blackberries
⅔ cup Spiced Vinegar (see page 139)
4½ cups warmed sugar (see page 7)

Tie the cloves, cinnamon sticks, and allspice berries in a cheesecloth bag and put in a large saucepan together with the blackberries and vinegar. Bring the mixture to a boil, then simmer gently, stirring occasionally, for about 30 minutes.

Strain the mixture through a nonmetallic sieve and return to the pan. Discard the bag. Over low heat, stir in the warmed sugar until it has dissolved, then continue to simmer, stirring as necessary, until well thickened.

Ladle the jelly into warm, clean, dry jars. Cover and seal (see pages 12–13). Store in a cool, dark, dry place for at least 3 weeks before eating.

Serving Suggestion
Serve with game, pork, turkey, or duck or add to casseroles made with them.

Right: Quick Savory Blackberry Jelly makes a delicious dressing for this sweet-sour Duck Salad.

Duck Salad with Blackberry Dressing

SERVES 4

4 duck breasts, 5–6 ounces each
sea salt
mixed salad greens, such as watercress, arugula, bibb lettuce, curly endive and baby spinach
flat-leaf parsley
1½ tablespoons red wine

1 tablespoon red wine vinegar
1 tablespoon Quick Savory Blackberry Jelly (see left)
about 1½ tablespoons sunflower seeds

Preheat the oven to 450°F.

Rub the duck breasts with salt, then score the skin with the point of a sharp knife. Put the breasts, skin side up, on a rack in a roasting pan and roast for 15 minutes.

Divide the salad greens and parsley among 4 plates.

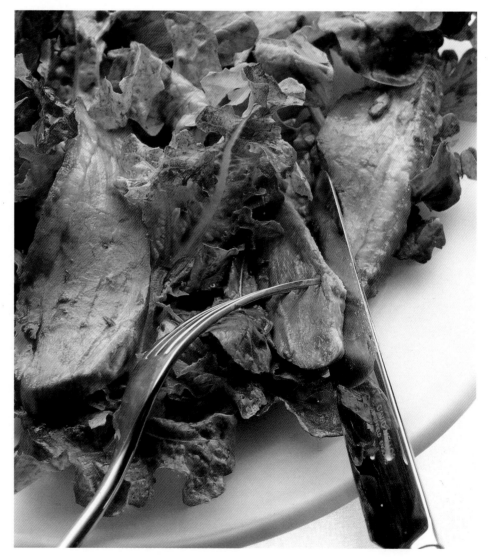

𝓑LACKBERRIES AND 𝓑LUEBERRIES

Transfer the duck to a warm plate and keep warm for about 10 minutes.

Tilt the roasting pan and spoon off the surplus fat, leaving behind the juices. Put the pan on the stove to caramelize the juices. Using a wooden spoon, stir in the wine and vinegar to dislodge the pan juices and bring to a boil for 1–2 minutes, stirring frequently.

Remove from the heat and stir in the jelly, then set aside. Cut the duck into strips and add them to the salad greens and sprinkle with the sunflower seeds.

Gently reheat the sauce in the roasting pan to dissolve the jelly, then bring to a boil. Pour over the duck and salad greens, toss lightly, and serve.

Blackberry and Apple Jelly with Thyme

You can vary the amount of thyme used in this recipe according to taste.

MAKES 4 CUPS

1½ pounds cooking apples
3 pounds blackberries
handful of fresh thyme sprigs
warmed sugar (see page 7)
thyme leaves (optional)

Coarsely chop the apples without peeling or coring them, then put them into a pan with the blackberries, thyme sprigs, and 2½ cups water. Bring to a boil, then simmer for 1 hour, stirring occasionally, until the fruit is soft.

Pour the contents of the pan into a scalded jelly bag suspended over a nonmetallic bowl and leave to strain, undisturbed, in a cool place for 8–12 hours.

Measure the strained juice and put into a pan with 2¼ cups warmed sugar for every 2½ cups juice. Heat gently, stirring, until the sugar has dissolved, then raise the heat and

boil vigorously for about 15 minutes or until setting point is reached (see page 17).

Remove from the heat and taste a little of the jelly – if the thyme flavor is not strong enough, leave to stand for 10–15 minutes, then stir in some thyme leaves. Ladle into warm, clean, dry jars. Cover, seal, and process (see pages 12–13). Leave overnight to set. Store in a cool, dark, dry place.

Blueberry Curd

With their sweet juiciness, blueberries are ideal candidates for making a fruit curd.

MAKES 1⅓ CUPS

8 ounces blueberries
¼ cup unsalted butter, diced
1¼ cups superfine sugar
3 large eggs, lightly beaten

Place the blueberries in a covered saucepan with 1 tablespoon water and cook gently, shaking the pan occasionally, until very soft (about 10 minutes). Press through a fine nonmetallic sieve into a heatproof nonmetallic bowl or the top of a double boiler, then stir in the butter and sugar and put over a saucepan of gently simmering water; do not allow the bottom of the bowl to sit in the water. Heat gently, stirring, until the sugar has dissolved and the butter has melted.

Strain in the eggs and continue to stir over gently simmering water until the curd thickens enough to coat the back of the spoon, which should take 30–40 minutes. Stir only occasionally at first, more frequently as the cooking progresses, then constantly toward the end so that the curd cooks evenly and does not curdle. The water must not boil.

Strain the curd into warm, clean, dry jars. Cover, seal, and process (see pages 12–13). Store in a cold, dark, dry place or the refrigerator. Refrigerate after opening.

Blueberry Jam

MAKES ABOUT 4⅔ CUPS

3 pounds blueberries
juice of 2 lemons
4 small fresh bay leaves
5 cups sugar
commercial liquid pectin or 1 cup pectin extract (see page 7)

Stir the blueberries, lemon juice, bay leaves, and half the sugar together in a nonmetallic bowl, crushing the berries slightly. Cover and leave in a cool place for 6–8 hours.

Transfer the contents of the bowl to a saucepan and add the pectin extract and remaining sugar (if using commercial pectin, follow the manufactuer's directions). Stir over low heat until the sugar has dissolved, then boil for 4 minutes or until setting point is reached (see page 17).

Remove from the heat, scoop out the bay leaves, and skim off any scum. Leave to stand for 10–15 minutes. Stir, then pour into warm, clean, dry jars. Cover, seal, and process (see pages 12–13). Leave overnight to set. Store in a cool, dark, dry place.

Below: Ripe blackberries.

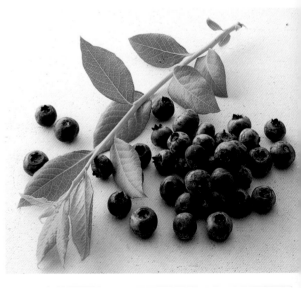

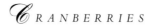
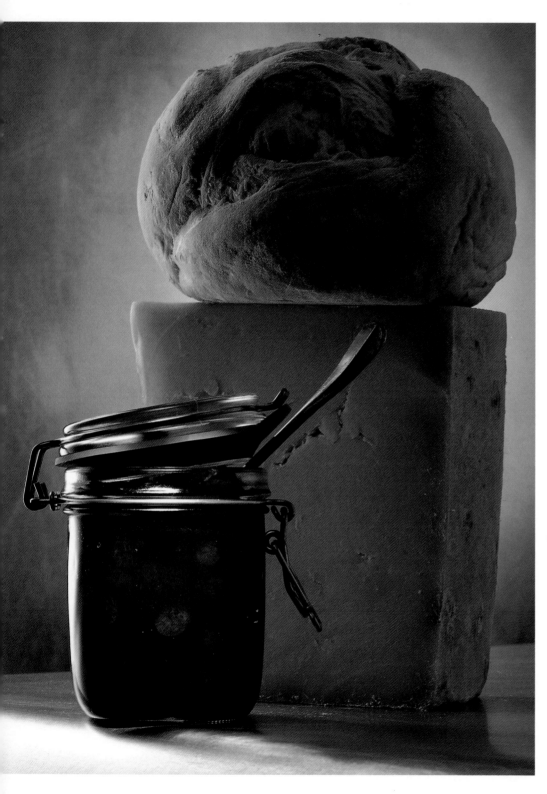

Cranberry Chutney

Bright red cranberries are too sour to eat raw, but once cooked, they can be transformed into a variety of delicious sauces and chutneys. This is a fresher, lighter chutney than many; I prefer to use white rather than brown sugar, as it keeps the color and flavor light.

MAKES ABOUT 3⅓ CUPS

1 pound cranberries
1 pound sweet apples, peeled, cored,
**   and chopped**
⅔ cup raisins
1 ounce fresh ginger, peeled and grated
grated zest of 1 orange
½ cinnamon stick
pinch of ground cloves
rock or sea salt
about 1¼ cups white sugar
scant 2 cups white wine vinegar or cider vinegar

Put all the ingredients into a large saucepan and heat gently, stirring, until the sugar has dissolved. Raise the heat and bring the contents of the pan to a boil, then simmer gently for about 30 minutes, stirring occasionally, until all the fruit is soft, the chutney is thick, and there is no free liquid.

  Spoon the chutney into warm, clean, dry jars making sure that you do not trap any air bubbles. Cover the chutney with acid-proof lids, seal, and process (see pages 12–13). Store in a cool, dark, dry place for at least 2 months before eating.

Left: Cranberry Chutney goes particularly well with good fresh bread and a variety of traditional hard cheeses.

𝒞RANBERRIES

Spiced Cranberry and Apple Sauce

Traditional pickling spices, tart fruit, vinegar, and sugar combine to make a fruity, sharp sauce that is good with pork and duck.

MAKES ABOUT 2⅔ CUPS

1 pound cranberries
8 ounces cooking apples, peeled, cored, and chopped
1¼ cups white wine vinegar
6 whole cloves
6 allspice berries
2 blades of mace
2 cinnamon sticks
1¾ cups warmed sugar (see page 7)

Put the cranberries, apples, and vinegar into a pan. Put the spices on a square of cheesecloth and tie into a bag with a long length of string. Tie the free end of the string to the handle of the pan so that the bag is resting on the fruit. Bring to a boil, then cover and simmer for 10 minutes or until the cranberries and apples are soft but retain their shape.

Remove the pan from the heat and stir in the warmed sugar. Heat gently, stirring, until

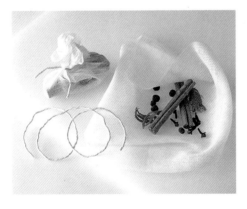

Preserving with spices: Tie spices in a piece of cheesecloth. The spices will flavor the preserve and the bag is easy to remove.

the sugar has dissolved, then simmer for about 20 minutes or until thickened.

Remove the pan from the heat. Discard the spice bag and pour the sauce into warm, clean, dry jars. Cover with acid-proof lids, seal, and process (see pages 12–13). Store the sauce in a cool, dark, dry place for 6–8 weeks before eating.

Quick Cranberry and Orange Jelly

This recipe is a jelly because it does not contain any pieces of fruit or seeds, yet it does not have the usual clarity of jellies. Because the cooked fruit is pressed through a sieve rather than left to strain for hours, the whole process is a much quicker one. Needless to say, this jelly goes well with Thanksgiving or Christmas roast turkey.

MAKES ABOUT 2⅔ CUPS

1 pound cranberries
grated zest of 1 orange
2¼ cups warmed sugar (see page 7)

Put the cranberries, orange zest, and 1¼ cups water in a large saucepan and bring to a boil over moderate heat, then simmer, stirring occasionally, for 10 minutes or until the cranberries pop and the mixture becomes a thick pulp.

Press the contents of the pan through a nonmetallic sieve.

Return the purée to the rinsed pan and add the warmed sugar. Heat gently, stirring, until the sugar has dissolved, then heat for about 5 minutes or until small bubbles just begin to appear around the edge of the pan.

Remove from the heat immediately and ladle into warm clean, dry jars. Cover, seal, and process (see pages 12–13). Leave overnight to set. Store the jelly in a cool, dark, dry place.

Cranberry Ketchup

Cranberry Ketchup makes a more than acceptable alternative to cranberry jelly with turkey.

MAKES ABOUT 2½–3¾ CUPS

2 pounds cranberries
8 ounces onions, chopped
⅔ cup white wine vinegar
1½ cups sugar
1 teaspoon salt
6 allspice berries
4 whole cloves
10 black peppercorns
2-inch piece cinnamon stick

Put the cranberries, onions, and 1¼ cups water in a large saucepan and bring to a boil, then simmer gently until the cranberries have burst and the onions are tender. Press through a fine nonmetallic sieve.

Return the purée to the rinsed pan with the vinegar, sugar, and salt. Tie the spices in a square of cheesecloth and add to the pan. Heat gently, stirring, until the sugar has dissolved. Raise the heat and bring to a boil, then simmer for about 15 minutes or until the sauce has the consistency of sour cream and there is no free liquid.

Remove the spice bag from the pan and discard. Pour the ketchup into warm, clean, dry bottles. Cover, seal, and process (see pages 12–13). Store in a cool, dark, dry place for 2–3 weeks before eating.

Serving Suggestion
Cranberry Ketchup is useful to have in reserve, as a couple of spoonfuls can be stirred into the cooking juices of roast turkey to make a quick gravy. It is also excellent for livening up many sauces and casseroles.

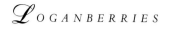

Loganberry Jam

For as long as I can remember, loganberries have been grown by my family, first by my grandparents and then by my mother. They always seemed to have been planted so that the berries would be difficult to reach, but that and the sharp prickles never deterred even small hands and arms from reaching for the plump, sweet fruit. Loganberries are particularly flavorful berries.

MAKES ABOUT 6⅓ CUPS

3 pounds loganberries
juice of ½ lemon
7 cups warmed sugar (see page 7)

Gently heat the loganberries and lemon juice in a covered heavy casserole in a very low oven until soft and thoroughly hot (45–60 minutes). Alternatively, gently heat the fruit and lemon juice in a large saucepan without any water until the juice runs, then simmer for about 15 minutes, stirring occasionally, until the fruit is very soft.

Transfer the contents of the casserole to a pan. Over low heat, gently stir in the sugar until it has dissolved. Raise the heat and boil vigorously for about 10 minutes or until setting point is reached (see page 17).

Remove from the heat and skim the scum from the surface with a slotted spoon. Leave to stand for 10–15 minutes. Stir and ladle into warm, clean, dry jars. Cover, seal, and process (see pages 12–13). Leave overnight to set. Store in a cool, dark, dry place.

Crisp Loganberry and Pear Phyllo Rolls

SERVES 4

generous ¼ cup Loganberry Jam
(see left)
¼ cup raisins

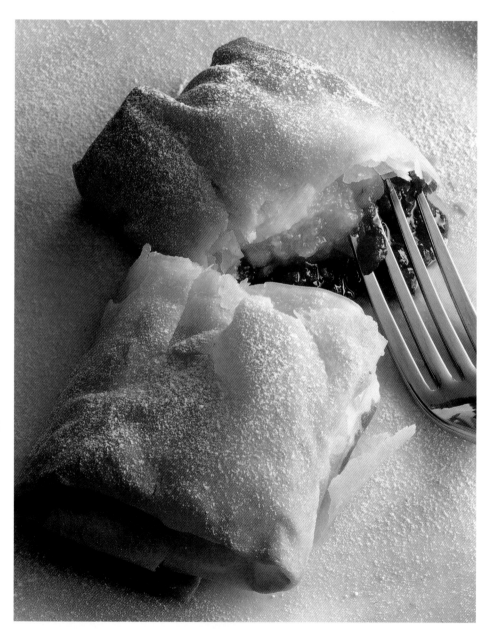

1 cup fresh bread crumbs
1 teaspoon ground cinnamon
1 large pear, peeled, cored, and quartered
4 sheets of phyllo pastry, each measuring about
12 inches × 7 inches
melted unsalted butter for brushing
sifted confectioners' sugar for dusting

Right: Crisp Loganberry and Pear Phyllo Rolls consist of individual plump cushions of fruit wrapped in a crunchy layer of pastry.

$\mathcal{R}$ASPBERRIES

Preheat the oven to 350°F. Lightly butter a baking sheet.

Mix together the loganberry jam, raisins, bread crumbs, and cinnamon.

Brush one sheet of phyllo pastry with melted butter, then fold it in half and brush again with butter. Spoon a quarter of the cranberry mixture along the edge nearest you and put a pear quarter on top. Fold the sides of the pastry over the filling, then roll up neatly. Transfer to the baking sheet, putting the seam side down. Repeat with the remaining filling, pastry, and pear quarters.

Brush each roll with melted butter and bake for 20–30 minutes or until pale golden. Serve the rolls either hot or cold dusted with confectioners' sugar.

Quick Uncooked Raspberry Jam

To gain the full benefit of this jam, which preserves the true fresh flavor of the fruit, use the most full-flavored berries you can find. Raspberries that are less than great in flavor can be boosted with *eau-de-vie de framboise* (raspberry eau-de-vie). Instead of adding kirsch to the fruit mixture, try flavoring the jam with rosewater. The jam is much softer than conventional boiled jams.

MAKES ABOUT 2⅔ CUPS

1 pound raspberries
2¼ cups superfine sugar
1 tablespoon kirsch (optional)

Preheat the oven to 325°F.

Put the raspberries and sugar in separate large heatproof bowls, cover, and put in the oven for 20–30 minutes or until very hot but not quite boiling.

Transfer the raspberries and sugar to a large bowl and stir together thoroughly using a wooden spoon. Stir in the kirsch if using, then spoon into warm, clean, dry jars. Cover, seal, and process (see pages 12–13). Store in a cool, dark, dry place for at least 1 month before eating.

Serving Suggestion
Serve over peaches, strawberries, or pears or eat with fresh ricotta or mascarpone cheese. Crisp almond cookies make a good companion to any of these.

Framboise

When genuine French liqueurs such as framboise and cassis are made, the fruit is macerated in molasses spirits for about 2 months before the juice is squeezed out, sweetened, and distilled. This is a much easier method, but the result is still delicious, both as a drink or poured over fruit or ice cream to create mouthwatering desserts.

MAKES 5 CUPS

1 pound raspberries
2½ cups brandy
about 1¾ cups sugar

Lightly crush the raspberries, then put them in a screw-top jar with the brandy. Close tightly and leave in a cool, dark, dry place for 2 months.

Strain the liqueur through a nonmetallic sieve lined with cheesecloth, measure the liquid, and stir in ¾ cup plus 2 tablespoons sugar for every 2½ cups. Cover and leave for 2 days, stirring occasionally to dissolve the sugar.

Pour the framboise into bottles, seal (see pages 12–13), and store in a cool, dark, dry place for at least 6 months before drinking.

Variations: *Crème de Cassis*
Follow the recipe above, simply substituting black currants for raspberries. Makes about 5 cups.
Crème de Mûres
Follow the recipe above, simply substituting blackberries for raspberries. Makes about 5 cups.

Serving Suggestion
Dilute with still or sparkling dry white wine; pour over fruit such as peaches, strawberries, or pears; pour over creamy desserts and ice cream.

Below (from left to right): Fresh loganberries and raspberries.

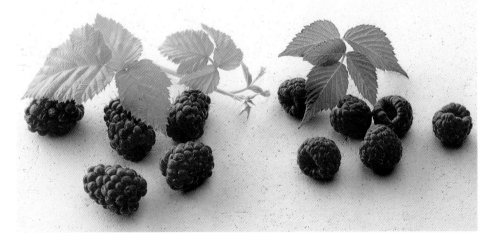

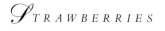
Strawberry Conserve

Making this preserve, which captures the true fresh flavor of strawberries and contains whole plump berries, doesn't take much time, although the method does stretch over 3 days.

MAKES ABOUT 4 CUPS

2¼ pounds strawberries, hulled
4½ cups warmed sugar (see page 7)
juice of 1 lemon or orange

Layer the strawberries and warmed sugar in a large saucepan, cover, and leave overnight in a cool place, by which time most of the sugar should have dissolved.

Gently heat the pan to dissolve any remaining sugar and draw the juice from the fruit; give an occasional gentle stir or shake the pan so that the fruit stays whole. Add the lemon or orange juice, raise the heat, and boil for 5 minutes.

Carefully pour the mixture into a non-metallic bowl, cover, and leave in a cool place for 2 days. Return to the pan, bring to a boil, and boil vigorously for 10 minutes. Remove from the heat and skim any scum from the surface with a slotted spoon. Leave to stand for 10–15 minutes. Stir and ladle into warm, clean, dry jars. Cover, seal, and process (see pages 12–13). Leave overnight to set. Store in a cool, dark, dry place.

Freezer Strawberry Jam

Freezer jams have a very soft set. If you add commercial liquid pectin or pectin extract as in this recipe, you will have a firmer set. Use containers that will neither react with the acid in the fruit nor crack when frozen. Freezer jams can be frozen for up to 6 months. Once thawed, they must be kept in the refrigerator, where they will keep for 2 or 3 days.

MAKES ABOUT 4 CUPS

2 pounds strawberries
2¼ cups sugar
commercial liquid pectin or ⅔ cup pectin extract (see page 7)
juice of 1 lemon

Place the strawberries in a nonmetallic bowl and crush with a wooden spoon. Stir in the pectin extract and sugar (if using commercial pectin, follow the manufacturer's directions). Then cover and place in an oven preheated to the lowest setting until warm but not hot. Remove the bowl and leave to stand for for 1 hour, stirring occasionally, until the sugar has dissolved.

Stir in the lemon juice, then pack into small freezer containers, leaving plenty of headroom to allow for expansion during freezing. Cover and seal (see pages 12–13).

Leave to stand at a cool temperature for 6 hours, then refrigerate for 24–48 hours or until jelled. Store in the freezer. Return to room temperature 1 hour before serving.

Serving Suggestion
Warm and pour over bread pudding; spoon over ice cream or eat with plain yogurt.

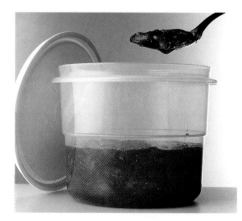

Freezer jams: These are not boiled, as ordinary jams are, so they have a softer set. They have a particularly fresh and delicious flavor.

Strawberry and Rhubarb Jam

I first tasted strawberries and rhubarb together in a pie filling and have since combined them in a jam.

MAKES ABOUT 6 CUPS

1 pound strawberries, halved if large
3 pounds rhubarb, cut into ½-inch lengths
7 cups warmed sugar (see page 7)
3 lemons, halved

Layer the fruit and sugar in a nonmetallic bowl. Squeeze the lemons, reserving the seeds and peels. Pour the juice over the fruit and sugar, cover, and leave in a cool place overnight.

Chop the lemon halves, then tie them in a cheesecloth bag with the seeds. Pour the fruit mixture into a large saucepan and add the cheesecloth bag. If the sugar has not dissolved, heat gently until it does. Bring quickly to a boil and boil vigorously for about 15 minutes, stirring as necessary, until setting point is reached (see page 17).

Remove from the heat and skim the scum from the surface with a slotted spoon. Discard the bag. Leave the jam to stand for 10–15 minutes. Stir and ladle into warm, clean, dry jars. Cover, seal, and process (see pages 12–13). Leave overnight to set. Store in a cool, dark, dry place.

Black Currant Jam

With its rich, full, fruity flavor and its strong, dark color, this black currant jam is one of my favorites.

MAKES ABOUT 7 CUPS

3 pounds black currants
10¼ cups warmed sugar (see page 7)

ℬLACK CURRANTS

Put the black currants in a pan with 5 cups water and bring to a boil. Lower the heat and simmer, stirring occasionally, for 45–60 minutes or until the fruit skins are soft and the water reduced by about one-third.

Over low heat, stir in the sugar until it has completely dissolved, then raise the heat and boil vigorously for 6–8 minutes, stirring occasionally, until setting point is reached (see page 17).

Remove the pan from the heat and skim the scum from the surface of the jam with a slotted spoon. Ladle into warm, clean, dry jars. Cover, seal, and process (see pages 12–13). Leave overnight to set. Store in a cool, dark, dry place.

Black Currant Cordial

When you make your own black currant cordial, there is no need to worry about it containing additives or preservatives.

MAKES ABOUT 3½ CUPS

4 pounds black currants
1¾–2¼ cups sugar
1½ lemons

Gently heat the black currants and 1¼ cups water in a large saucepan for about 20 minutes, crushing the black currants occasionally with a wooden spoon.

Press the contents of the pan through a nonmetallic sieve. Measure the juice and pour it back into the rinsed pan. Add 1¼–1½ cups sugar and the juice of 1 lemon for every 2½ cups juice and heat gently, stirring, until the sugar has dissolved. Raise the heat and boil for 1 minute.

Skim the scum from the surface with a slotted spoon, then pour the cordial into warm, clean, dry bottles, leaving ½ inch of headspace. Cover, then loosen the lid by half a turn. Process in a boiling water bath (see page 13) for 25 minutes. Remove the bottles from the water bath and tighten the lids immediately. Store in a cool, dark, dry place for up to 6 months.

Serving Suggestion
As well as using as the base for drinks (try adding 1 or 2 crushed mint leaves to drinks), black currant cordial can be poured over pears or ice cream and stirred into crème fraîche or thick yogurt. A decoration of mint looks particularly enticing.

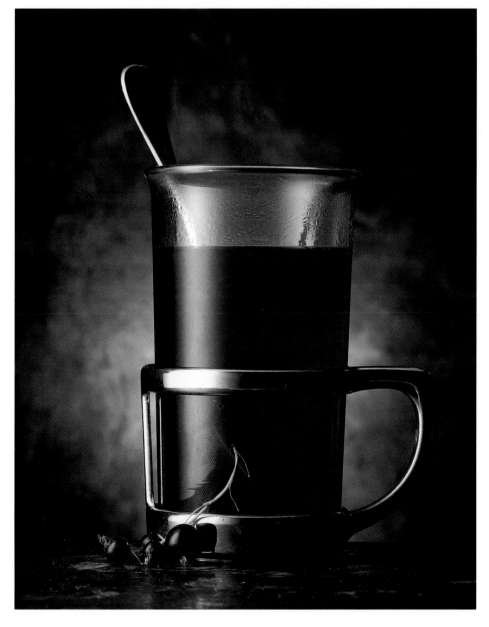

Left: Black Currant Cordial makes a deliciously refreshing summertime drink.

Spiced Red Currant Jelly with Drambuie

This is an ideal way of rescuing flavorless commercial red currant jelly. The spices continue to flavor the jelly after it is put into jars, so if you keep the jelly very long, you may want to remove the cinnamon and perhaps the cloves after a while (gently warming the jelly is the best way to do this). Pink peppercorns are not related to black peppercorns and have more of an aromatic, pine flavor than a peppery one.

MAKES ABOUT 1 CUP

thinly pared zest of 1 lemon, cut into fine shreds
12-ounce jar red currant jelly
juice of 1 lemon
3 tablespoons Drambuie
seeds from 2 cardamom pods, crushed
4 whole cloves
1 cinnamon stick
¼–½ teaspoon pink peppercorns
freshly ground black pepper

Add the lemon shreds to a small saucepan of boiling water and boil for 10 minutes. Drain and refresh under running cold water. Drain and dry on paper towels.

Gently melt the red currant jelly with the lemon juice and shreds and 2 tablespoons Drambuie, stirring until smooth. Add the spices and pepper and boil vigorously for 4 minutes or until setting point is reached (see page 17).

Remove from the heat, add the remaining Drambuie, and leave to stand for 10–15 minutes. Ladle the jelly into a warm, clean, dry jar. Cover, seal, and process (see pages 12–13). Leave overnight to set. Store in a cool, dark, dry place.

Serving Suggestion
Serve with cold ham or cold roast pork or turkey; eat French style with plain soft cheeses or plain crisp cookies for dessert.

Superlative Red Currant Jelly

This easy no-cook recipe is my favorite way of making red currant jelly, as it preserves the clean, fresh taste of the fruit. It has a lighter set than other red currant jellies; just how runny it is will depend on the amount of pectin and acid in the currants. (If you would like a firmer set, boil the juice and dissolved sugar until setting point is reached.) Unfortunately, this jelly does not keep as long as some jellies, so it's one of the preserves I use first rather than one I hang on to for months. If you don't have somewhere nice and cool to keep it, the warmest part of the refrigerator, such as the vegetable drawer, is probably the best place.

3–3½ pounds red currants
2½ cups warmed sugar (see page 7)

Purée the red currants by pressing them through a nonmetallic sieve or blending them and then pouring them through the sieve, then pour into a scalded jelly bag set over a large nonmetallic bowl and leave to strain, undisturbed, in a cool place for 8–12 hours.

Preheat the oven to low to moderate heat – the exact temperature is not important. Measure the strained juice into a heatproof bowl and add 1¾ cups sugar for every 2½ cups juice. Put the bowl in the oven until the mixture is really hot. Pour the red currant juice into a warm, deep saucepan and vigorously stir with a wooden spoon until the sugar has dissolved and the mixture has slightly stiffened.

Remove the pan from the heat and skim any scum from the surface with a slotted spoon. Immediately ladle the jelly into warm, clean, dry jars. Cover, seal, and process (see pages 12–13). Leave overnight to set. Store in a cool, dark, dry place.

Red Currant Gin

MAKES ABOUT 2 QUARTS

1¼ pounds red currants
1½ cups superfine sugar
3½ cups gin

Crush the red currants with the sugar, then transfer the mixture to a jar. Pour in the gin, cover, seal, and shake the jar. Leave in a cool, dark, dry place for 3 months, shaking the jar every day for 4 weeks, then only occasionally.

Strain the gin if desired, and pour into clean bottles. Alternatively, serve the gin by pouring it through a cheesecloth-lined nonmetallic sieve, and top up the jar with more fruit and sugar as the level goes down. Sieve to serve.

Variations: *Raspberry Gin*
Follow the recipe, substituting raspberries, but do not crush the berries. Simply put all the ingredients in a jar. If available, use vanilla-flavored sugar. Makes about 2 quarts.
Blackberry Gin
Use ripe fruit and follow the recipe, simply substituting blackberries for red currants. There is no need to crush the berries. Makes about 2 quarts.

Serving Suggestion
Serve after meals or as an evening warmer.

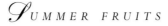

Summer Fruit Compote

In France this is known as *confiture de vieux garçons* (bachelors' jam). I suppose it is so named because it is extremely easy to make, requires no cooking, and is alcoholic. I'm sure plenty of bachelors will be offended by these implications; I'm equally sure that there are many nonbachelors to whom this recipe will appeal.

MAKES ABOUT 2 CUPS

1 pound prepared summer fruits, such as strawberries, raspberries, loganberries, and red and black currants
¾ cup plus 2 tablespoons superfine sugar
1¼–1⅔ cup kirsch

Layer the fruit and sugar in a clean, dry preserving jar or other wide-mouthed jar and leave for 2 hours.

Pour enough kirsch into the jar to cover the fruit. Cover and seal the jar (see pages 12–13). Store in a cool, dark, dry place for at least 1 month before eating, turning the jar upside down every week or so.

Red Summer Fruits Preserve

Capture the taste and memories of summer with this delicious and attractive preserve. I like to use raspberry eau-de-vie to intensify and fortify the flavor. Raspberry or cherry brandy will also add color and sweetness.

MAKES ABOUT 5 CUPS

1½ pounds raspberries
6 tablespoons lemon juice
⅔ cup freshly squeezed orange juice
7 cups warmed sugar (see page 7)
2 pounds mixed red summer fruits, such as loganberries, red currants, strawberries, and pitted red cherries
¼ cup raspberry eau-de-vie (see above)

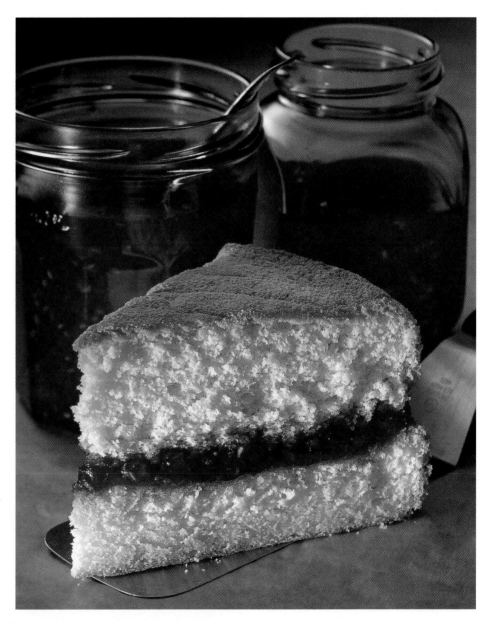

In a saucepan, gently cook the raspberries in the lemon and orange juices for 5–10 minutes or until soft. Press through a non-metallic sieve and return to the rinsed pan.

Stir in the warmed sugar over low heat until dissolved, then add the remaining fruit, raise the heat, and boil vigorously for 10–15 minutes, stirring as necessary, until setting point is reached.

Above: Red Summer Fruits Preserve makes an appropriately light filling for a light sponge cake.

Remove from the heat, skim any scum from the surface, and stir in the eau-de-vie. Leave for 10 minutes, then stir and ladle into warm, clean, dry jars. Cover, seal, and process (see pages 12–13). Leave overnight to set. Store in a cool, dark, dry place.

Gooseberry Sauce

Although customarily made with brown sugar, this sauce can be made with white, in which case it can be served with grilled mackerel or deep-fried Camembert.

MAKES ABOUT 5 CUPS

2 pounds green gooseberries
2 cups Spiced Vinegar (see page 139)
3⅓ cups warmed demerara or light
    brown sugar (see page 7)
1 teaspoon ground cinnamon

Put the fruit and vinegar in a saucepan and bring to a boil, then simmer for 10–15 minutes or until tender. Purée in a blender or press through a fine nonmetallic sieve, then return the purée to the rinsed pan.

Add the warmed sugar and the cinnamon to the puréed gooseberries and heat, stirring, until the sugar has dissolved. Raise the heat and simmer for 10–15 minutes, stirring frequently, to make a thick sauce.

Pour the sauce into warm, clean, dry jars. Cover, seal, and process (see pages 12–13). Store in a cool, dark, dry place.

Roast Pork Loin with Gooseberry Sauce

SERVES 4

2 tablespoons fresh white bread crumbs
about ½ cup Gooseberry Sauce
    (see above)
1½ pounds boneless pork loin
salt and freshly ground black pepper
olive oil for rubbing pork
¾–1 cup medium-bodied dry white wine

Preheat the oven to 350°F.

In a bowl, combine the bread crumbs with 2 tablespoons gooseberry sauce.

Unroll the pork loin, then season the inside with salt and pepper. Spread thinly with the

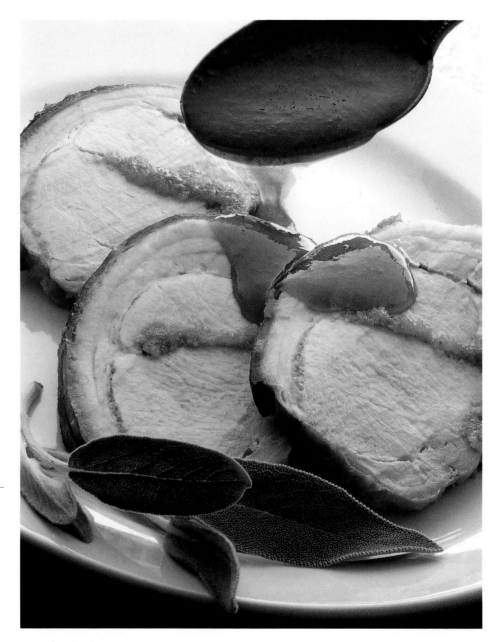

gooseberry sauce mixture. Reroll the loin and tie into shape. Rub olive oil over the outside and season with pepper.

Place the pork in a roasting pan and roast for 30 minutes per pound of meat plus 30 minutes extra.

Transfer the pork to a warm plate and keep warm. Spoon the fat from the roasting

Above: Roast Pork Loin is both stuffed and served with Gooseberry Sauce.

pan, then stir the white wine into the pan juices. Boil vigorously for a few minutes until most of the white wine has evaporated, then stir in the remaining gooseberry sauce. Season and serve with the pork.

*G*OOSEBERRIES AND *F*IGS

Gooseberry and Raspberry Jam

Raspberry and gooseberry jams are notorious for their seeds, so here is a smooth, seed- and skin-free jam. (This does mean that the yield is less than if the fruit were left unsieved, which you can, of course, do.) It is also a very fruity jam, as the fruit is heated without any water until tender in a low oven and commercial liquid pectin or pectin extract is used to minimize the boiling-to-set time (you will need to stir the jam frequently during this time).

MAKES ABOUT 7½ CUPS

2 pounds ripe gooseberries
1½ pounds raspberries
about 7 cups warmed sugar (see page 7)
commercial liquid pectin or 1 cup pectin extract
  (see page 7)

Put the fruit in a heavy heatproof dish, cover, and place in an oven set to the lowest temperature for about 2 hours, mashing the fruit occasionally with a wooden spoon, until it has softened.

  Press the fruit through a nonmetallic sieve with a wooden spoon, pressing down well on the skins, seeds, and pulp to push through as much extract as possible.

  Weigh the extract and put into a pan with an equal weight of sugar and ⅔ cup pectin extract for each 2 pounds puréed fruit (if using commercial pectin, follow the manufacturer's directions). Heat gently, stirring, until the sugar has dissolved. Raise the heat and boil vigorously for at least 4 minutes, stirring frequently, until setting point is reached (see page 17).

  Remove from the heat and skim any scum from the surface with a slotted spoon. Leave to stand for 10–15 minutes, then ladle it into warm, clean, dry jars. Cover, seal, and process (see pages 12–13). Leave overnight to set. Store in a cool, dark, dry place.

Fig Conserve

This conserve has a fresh, fruity taste because it is cooked briefly, which preserves the delicate scented flavor. The low sugar content makes it quite runny and means it does not keep long, so use it within 3 months. Choose fruit that is not too ripe.

MAKES ABOUT 5 CUPS

2 lemons
2 whole cloves
2 pounds figs, quartered
2¼ cups warmed sugar (see page 7)

Grate the zest from the lemons and squeeze out the juice, reserving the seeds. Tie the seeds and the cloves in a square of cheesecloth with a long piece of string. Tie the other end of the string to the handle of a pan so that the bag is suspended just above the bottom of the pan. Add the lemon juice, figs, and ⅔ cup water to the pan and simmer for about 15 minutes or until the figs are tender. Remove the cheesecloth bag.

  Over low heat, stir in the warmed sugar and the lemon zest until the sugar has dissolved. Raise the heat and boil vigorously, stirring occasionally, for about 40 minutes or until thick and syrupy.

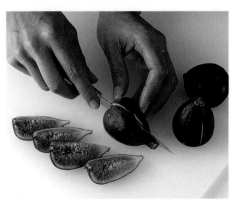

Preparing figs: Quarter figs lengthwise to display the attractive deep red interiors to their best advantage.

  Remove from the heat and skim the scum from the surface with a slotted spoon. Leave the conserve to stand for 10–15 minutes. Stir gently, then ladle into warm, clean, dry jars. Cover, seal, and process (see pages 12–13). Leave overnight to set. Store in a cool, dark, dry place. Refrigerate the conserve after opening.

Spiced Figs

This sweet-sour-spicy treat is ideal for using up figs that are not good enough to eat raw.

MAKES ABOUT 3 CUPS

1¼ cups superfine sugar
2 tablespoons clear honey
1¾ cups white wine vinegar
3 whole cloves
6 black peppercorns
2 cinnamon sticks
½-inch piece of fresh ginger, thinly sliced
3 allspice berries
pared zest of 1 lemon
scant 2 cups thickly sliced ripe but firm figs

Gently heat the sugar, honey, and vinegar together in a large saucepan, stirring, until the sugar has dissolved. Add the spices and lemon zest and boil for 1½ minutes. Remove the pan from the heat and add the figs. Return to the heat and bring to a boil, then simmer for 1 minute, pushing the fruit under the vinegar.

  Carefully pour the figs, spices, and vinegar into a nonmetallic bowl, cover, and leave to stand overnight.

  Using a slotted spoon, pack the fig slices tightly into a clean, dry jar.

  Boil the spiced vinegar for 15 minutes or until reduced to ⅔ cup. Pour into the jar, cover immediately with an acid-proof lid, seal, and process (see pages 12–13). Store in a cool, dark, dry place for at least 1 week before using.

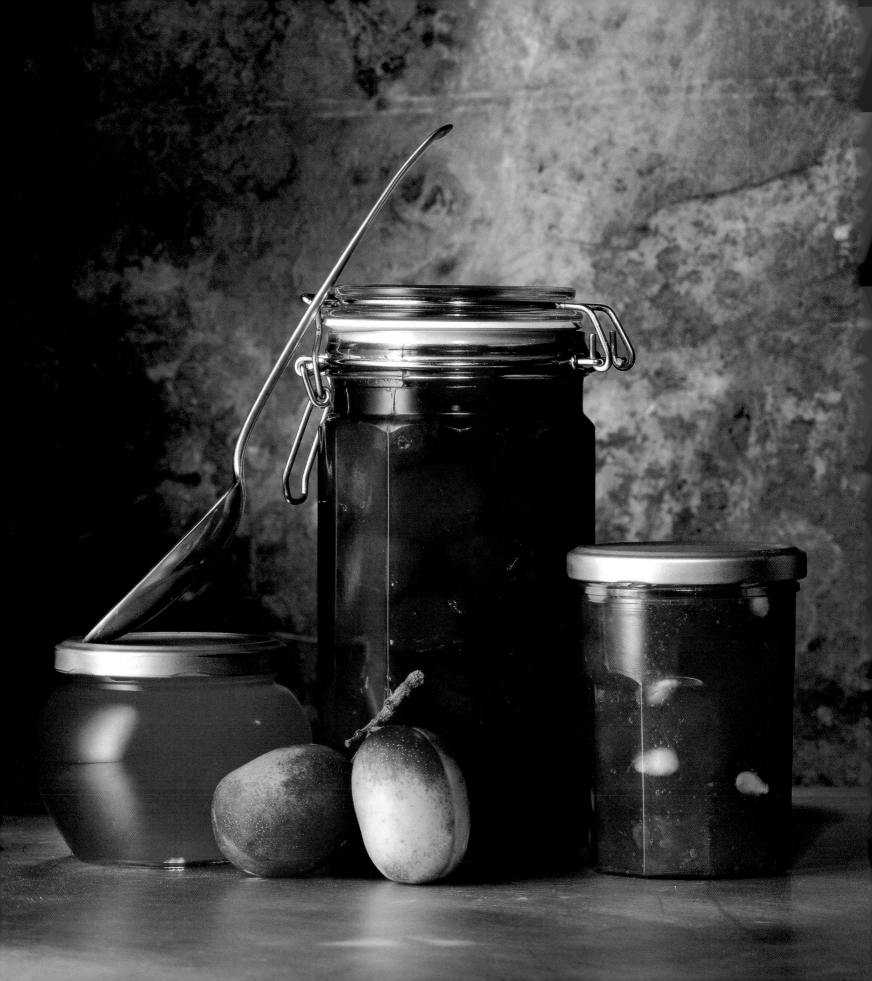

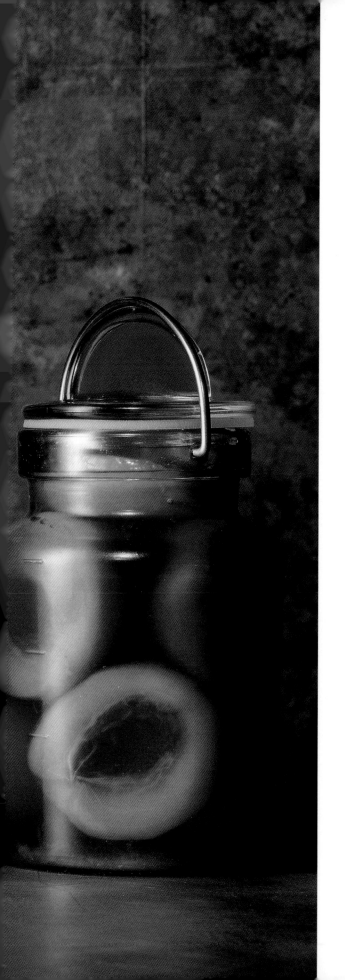

$\mathscr{S}$TONE $\mathscr{F}$RUITS

Stone fruits come from places as diverse as the orchards of America and the English countryside, the humid regions of southern India, and the warm terraces of the Mediterranean coast. Their enormous variety runs from exotic luscious mangoes to commonplace peaches and plums. In the United States, cherries inaugurate the stone-fruit year in May, followed by apricots, peaches, and nectarines as the summer progresses. Then come the plums. Fresh dates, mainly from California and Israel, are picked in the autumn but can be stored, so that they are available year round. Mangoes, too, are always in season somewhere in the world as different varieties come into season at different times. Although guavas have seeds, not stones, I have included a recipe for Guava Jelly (see page 109) in this chapter because it seemed the most appropriate place.

Left (from left to right): Plum Jelly, Spiced Plums, Apricot and Amaretto Conserve, and Nectarines in White Wine Syrup.

Chunky Apricot Chutney

This chunky chutney (the apricots are not cooked down) is fruity, mild, and refined.

MAKES 3⅓–4 CUPS

2¼ pounds ripe apricots, halved and pitted
⅔ cup raisins
1 onion, finely chopped
2–3 garlic cloves, very finely chopped
1 teaspoon coriander seeds, crushed
1¼ teaspoons grated fresh ginger
2 tablespoons sea salt
1½ cups light brown sugar
1¼ cups white wine vinegar

Put all the ingredients in a large saucepan and heat gently, stirring, until the sugar has dissolved. Raise the heat and boil, stirring occasionally, until the apricots are completely soft but not disintegrating.

Using a slotted spoon, transfer the apricots to warm, clean, dry jars and keep warm in a low oven.

Boil the liquid remaining in the pan until it becomes a thick syrup. Ladle into the jars, cover with acid-proof lids, and process (see pages 12–13). Store in a cool, dark, dry place for 1 month before eating.

Apricots in Cointreau

MAKES ABOUT 1½ QUARTS

1½ pounds large ripe, well-flavored apricots
1¾ cups superfine sugar
1¼ cups Cointreau
about 1 cup brandy or whiskey

Prick the apricots all over with a large embroidery needle or round toothpick, then layer them with the sugar in a clean, dry jar.

Mix together the Cointreau and brandy and pour into the jar to cover the fruit. Rotate the jar to dislodge any air bubbles, then seal and shake the jar (see pages 12–13).

Store in a cool, dark, dry place for at least 2 months before eating; shake the jar occasionally during the first week or so until the sugar has completely dissolved.

Fresh Apricot Jam

You need to use top-quality apricots for jam making. Any fruits that are woolly and lacking in flavor will make a poor-quality jam. Fruit that is not ripe enough to eat can, of course, be used. A warm, glowing sheen indicates a good flavor.

MAKES ABOUT 4 CUPS

2 pounds well-flavored apricots
juice of 1 small lemon
1 teaspoon grated lemon zest
4½ cups warmed sugar (see page 7)

Halve the apricots, reserving several of the pits. Crack the reserved pits with a nutcracker, rolling pin, or hammer. Remove the kernels and blanch them in boiling water for 1–2 minutes. Drain the kernels and slip off the skins.

Put the kernels into a large saucepan with the apricots, lemon juice and zest, and

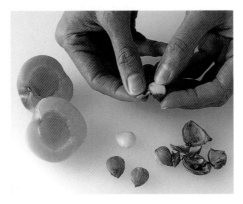

Preparing apricot kernels: Blanch the kernels in boiling water and drain. The skins should now slip off quite easily.

¾ cup water. Bring to a boil, then simmer for about 10–20 minutes or until tender.

Over low heat, stir in the warmed sugar until it has dissolved. Raise the heat and boil the contents of the pan vigorously, stirring occasionally, for about 15 minutes or until setting point is reached (see page 17).

Remove the pan from the heat and skim any scum from the surface with a slotted spoon. Leave the jam to stand for 10–15 minutes. Stir gently, then ladle the jam into warm, clean, dry jars. Cover, seal, and process (see pages 12–13). Leave overnight to set. Store in a cool, dark, dry place.

Apricot and Amaretto Conserve

MAKES ABOUT 2⅔ CUPS

1½ pounds fresh apricots
3½ cups vanilla sugar (see page 134)
3 tablespoons amaretto liqueur

Halve the apricots and remove the pits. Crack the pits with a rolling pin or hammer. Remove the kernels and blanch them in boiling water for 1–2 minutes. Drain and slip off the skins.

Layer the apricots and sugar in a nonmetallic bowl, cover, and leave overnight in a cool place, by which time most of the sugar should have dissolved.

Transfer the contents of the bowl to a large saucepan, add ⅔ cup water and the kernels, and heat gently, stirring, until any remaining sugar has dissolved. Raise the heat and boil vigorously for 15–20 minutes, stirring occasionally, until slightly thickened.

Remove from the heat. Skim any scum off the surface, then stir in the amaretto and leave for 10–15 minutes. Stir and ladle into warm, clean, dry jars. Cover, seal, and process (see pages 12–13). Leave overnight to set. Store in a cool, dark, dry place.

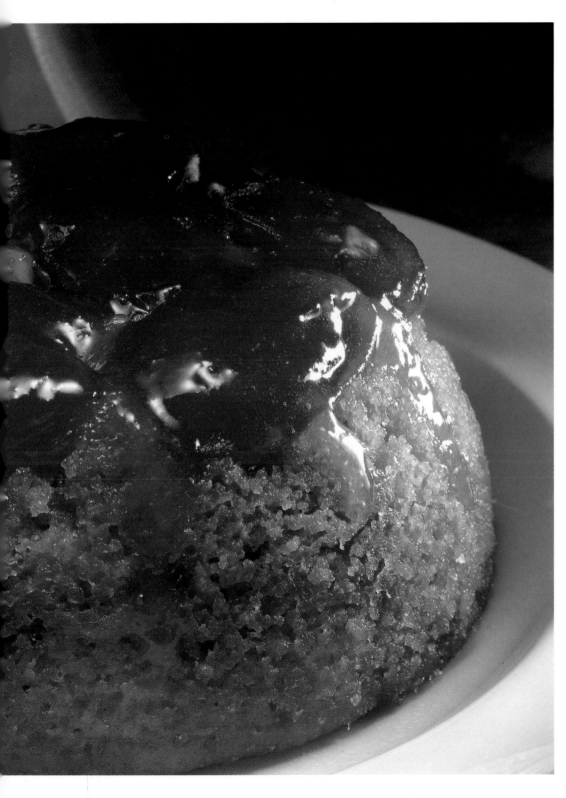

Light and Lovely Apricot Pudding

SERVES 4

Apricot and Amaretto Conserve (see page 96)
1½ tablespoons lemon juice
6 tablespoons butter, diced
1½ cups fresh white bread crumbs
generous ¼ teaspoon baking soda
3 tablespoons self-rising flour
⅓ cup demerara or raw sugar
2 large eggs, lightly beaten

Line the bottom of a buttered 2½–3 cup pudding mold with apricot halves from the conserve, placed cut sides up.

In a small saucepan, gently heat ¼ cup of the jelly from the conserve with the lemon juice and butter until the butter has melted.

Meanwhile, mix together the dry ingredients in a bowl. Stir in the butter mixture, then slowly pour in the eggs, mixing thoroughly. Spoon into the mold, taking care not to dislodge the apricots.

Make a fold across the center of a piece of buttered foil and place it loosely over the basin to allow the pudding to rise. Tie the foil in place with string around the mold rim and use the string to form a loose handle across the top of the foil. Put the mold in a steaming basket. Cover and place over a saucepan of boiling water and steam for about 1¾ hours or until the pudding is just set in the center.

Lift the mold out of the basket. Remove the string and foil. Run a knife around the sides of the mold to loosen the pudding, place a plate over the top, then turn the mold upside down. Serve warm with light cream, ice cream, or vanilla custard.

Left: Apricot and Amaretto Conserve is used to top Light and Lovely Apricot Pudding.

Apricot Brandy

MAKES ABOUT 3½ CUPS

12 large ripe, well-flavored apricots
1¼ cups superfine sugar
2½ cups brandy

Halve the apricots, reserving the pits. Cut the flesh into small pieces and put into a jar. Crack the pits with a nutcracker, rolling pin, or hammer. Remove the kernels, blanch them in boiling water for 1–2 minutes, then drain and slip off the skins (see page 96).

Add the kernels to the jar with the sugar. Pour in the brandy, then seal the jar and shake to dissolve the sugar.

Store in a cool, dark, dry place for 2 months before using, shaking the jar every couple of days. Strain off the brandy and pour into clean, dry bottles. Cover and seal (see pages 12–13). Eat the fruit separately.

Variation: *Cherry Brandy*
Trim the stems, if necessary, from 1 pound cherries to ¼ inch of the fruit. Prick the cherries well with a large embroidery needle or round toothpick and layer in a wide-mouthed jar with 6 tablespoons sugar. Pour in the brandy and proceed as above. Makes about 3½ cups.

Apricot Cordial

Use a fairly good-quality brandy for this recipe, as a less expensive one will ruin the cordial; white rum, gin, or vodka can be substituted. The strained apricots can be eaten as they are, used to fill crêpes, or made into a mousse or soufflé.

MAKES ABOUT 7 CUPS

9 ounces well-flavored dried apricot halves,
  coarsely chopped
2¼ cups dry white wine
¼ cup clear honey
⅔ cup brandy

Leave the apricots to macerate in the wine in a covered nonmetallic bowl for about 12 hours.

Transfer the contents of the bowl to a large saucepan and bring slowly to the simmering point. Stir in the honey until it has dissolved, then remove the pan from the heat, cover, and leave to cool.

Pour the contents of the pan into the bowl in which the apricots were macerated, cover, and leave in a cool place (but not the refrigerator) for 3 days, stirring occasionally.

Strain off the liquid and stir in the brandy. Pour into clean, dry bottles. Cover and seal (see pages 12–13). Store in a cool, dark, dry place for 2 months before drinking.

Serving Suggestion
As well as being a drink, this cordial is wonderful stirred into any fresh or dried fruit salad, over ice cream, with crêpes or waffles, and with freshly baked tarte tatin.

Nectarine Conserve

Here is an elegant, delicately flavored conserve to make in the height of summer, when nectarines are at their most succulent, sun-ripened best. Add a couple of spoonfuls or so of an orange liqueur or brandy if desired after removing the cooked conserve from the heat.

MAKES ABOUT 4 CUPS

2½ pounds ripe but firm nectarines
3⅓ cups warmed sugar (see page 7)
2 tablespoons lime juice

Peel the nectarines, reserving the skins. Halve and pit the fruit and layer the fruit with the sugar in a nonmetallic bowl. Cover and leave overnight, by which time most of the sugar will have dissolved.

Put the nectarine skins in a large saucepan, just cover with water, and boil until the water is reduced to a thin layer at the bottom of the pan. Press the contents of the pan through a nonmetallic sieve into another pan.

Pour the contents of the bowl into the pan, add the lime juice, and heat gently, stirring, until any remaining sugar has dissolved. Raise the heat and boil vigorously for 15–20 minutes or until slightly thickened.

Remove from the heat and leave to stand for 10–15 minutes or until the nectarines remain suspended in the syrup when stirred. Ladle into warm, clean, dry jars, taking care not to trap any air bubbles. Cover, seal, and process (see pages 12–13). Leave overnight to set. Store in a cool, dark, dry place.

Nectarine Butter

Simmering nectarines into a fruit butter really concentrates their flavor to make a memorable teatime or breakfast spread.

MAKES ABOUT 1⅓ CUPS

2 pounds ripe nectarines, peeled, pitted,
  and chopped
warmed sugar (see page 7)

Gently simmer the nectarines in 2 cups water, stirring occasionally, until soft. Press the fruit through a nonmetallic sieve with a wooden spoon.

Measure the purée and return to the rinsed pan. Stir in 10 tablespoons sugar for every 1 cup purée and stir over low heat until the sugar has dissolved. Raise the heat and boil for 30–45 minutes, stirring occasionally at first, then more frequently until the stirring is constant and the mixture resembles sour cream.

Spoon into warm, clean, dry jars; do not trap any air bubbles. Cover, seal, and process (see pages 12–13). Store the butter in a cool, dark, dry place for a few days before eating.

*N*ECTARINES

Freezer Nectarine Jam

MAKES ABOUT 3⅔ CUPS

**2 pounds ripe nectarines, peeled, pitted,
and coarsely chopped
commercial liquid pectin or ⅔ cup pectin extract
4½ cups sugar
juice of 1 lemon**

Thoroughly mix the nectarines, pectin extract, sugar, and lemon juice together in a nonmetallic bowl and place in an oven set to the lowest temperature to warm through gently (if using commercial pectin, follow the manufacturer's instructions). Remove from the oven, cover, and leave for 8 hours, stirring occasionally until you are sure all the sugar has dissolved.

Ladle into freezer plastic containers, leaving a good headspace to allow for expansion during freezing, then cover and put in the refrigerator for 24–48 hours or until the jam sets. Freeze for up to 6 months.

Bring the jam to room temperature 1 hour before serving. This jam will keep in the refrigerator for up to 2 days after opening.

Nectarines in White Wine Syrup

While this recipe does not demand a really good wine, do not use a thin, acidic one. If you like, you can add a small bunch of scented geranium leaves or lemon balm or some scented rose petals in place of the orange peel.

MAKES 5⅓ CUPS

**1¾ cups sugar
2 strips of orange peel
3 cups dry white wine
12 ripe but firm nectarines, peeled and halved
brandy**

In a large saucepan, gently heat the sugar and orange peel in the wine, stirring, until the sugar has dissolved. Bring just to the simmering point and simmer gently for about 8 minutes.

Add the nectarine halves to the syrup, in batches if necessary, and poach for 10 minutes or until tender.

Using a slotted spoon, pack the fruit into warm, clean, dry jars. Boil the syrup for 1 minute, remove the orange peel, and pour the syrup over the fruit. Add brandy to cover the nectarines. Cover and seal (see pages 12–13). Store in a cool, dark, dry place for 1 month before using.

Serving Suggestion
Serve lightly chilled, topped with thick yogurt, whipped cream, or mascarpone cheese and sprinkled with toasted sliced almonds; to top a tart filled with crème pâtissière; with almond crêpes.

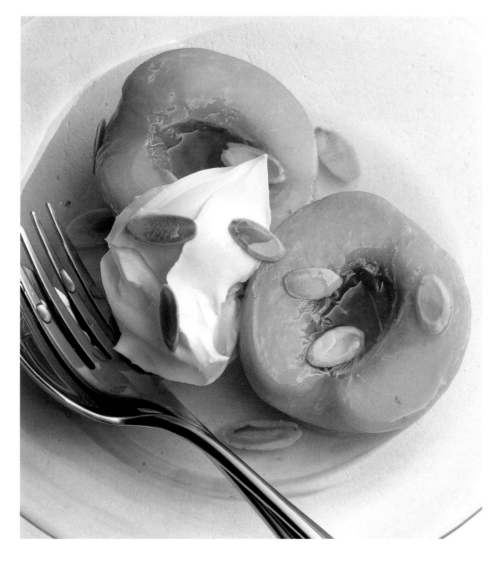

Left: Nectarines in White Wine Syrup are delicious served slightly chilled with mascarpone cheese and toasted sliced almonds.

Peach Spread

For this spread to be at its best you need to use ripe peaches that have basked in hot, clear sunshine until they are bursting with flavor. The aroma and flavor of peaches capture the essence of summer, and make this spread a real indulgence on a gray winter's day. An added bonus is that this recipe needs less boiling time than some other spreads.

MAKES ABOUT 1⅔ CUPS

2 pounds peaches
juice of 1 lemon
warmed sugar (see page 7)

Halve, pit, and slice the peaches without peeling them. Crack a few of the pits with a nutcracker, rolling pin, or hammer and remove the kernels. Blanch the kernels in boiling water for 1–2 minutes, then slip off the skins (see page 96).

Put the peaches, kernels, and lemon juice in a pan. Add water to just cover and bring to a boil, then simmer gently, covered, for about 20 minutes or so, or until the peaches are very soft.

Pour the contents of the pan into a scalded jelly bag suspended over a nonmetallic bowl and leave to strain, undisturbed, in a cool place for 8–12 hours.

Measure the juice and add 1¾ cups sugar for every 2½ cups juice. Heat gently, stirring, until the sugar has dissolved, then simmer gently for 40–45 minutes, stirring frequently, until the mixture is so thick and dry that the spoon leaves a clean line when drawn through it.

Spoon into warm, clean, dry jars or lightly oiled decorative molds. Cover, seal, and process (see pages 12–13). Store the spread in a cool, dark, dry place for at least 2–3 months before eating.

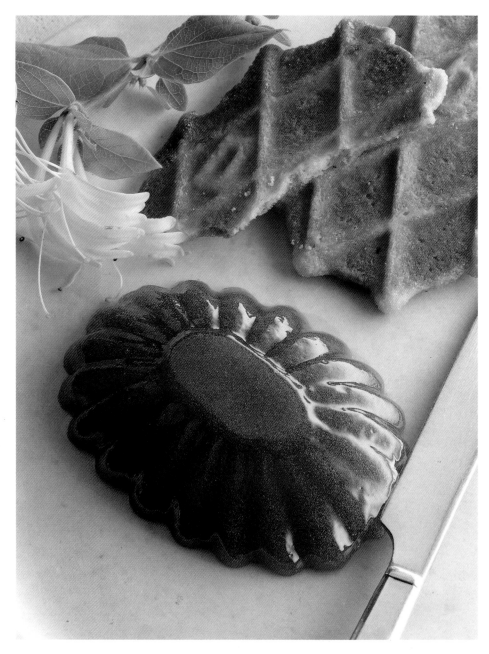

Serving Suggestion
Serve Peach Spread with mascarpone cheese and crisp almond cookies to make an instant dessert; serve on fresh, crusty bread for a delicious breakfast.

Above: This golden Peach Spread captures the heady scents of a summer's day.

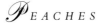

Peach and Raspberry Jam

Peaches and raspberries make a beautiful duo, as immortalized by the great chef Escoffier's Pêches Melba, created in honor of the opera singer Dame Nelly Melba.

MAKES ABOUT 6 CUPS

2 pounds 10 ounces peaches
2 tablespoons lemon juice
2¼ pounds raspberries
7 cups warmed sugar (see page 7)

Peel the peaches and put the skins on a square of cheesecloth. Halve the peaches and extract the pits. Crack the pits with a nutcracker, rolling pin, or hammer and remove the kernels. Add the kernels to the peach skins and tie the cheesecloth into a bag. Put ½ cup water and the lemon juice into a large saucepan. Chop the peaches, add to the pan, and tie the loose end of the cheesecloth bag string onto the pan handle so that it is suspended in the mixture. Bring the mixture to a boil, lower the heat, and simmer for about 20 minutes or until the peaches are soft.

Remove the pan from the heat and, using a slotted spoon, lift out the cheesecloth bag and press it firmly with the back of a metal spoon so that the juices run into the pan. Add the raspberries to the pan and return it to the heat, then simmer for 5 minutes.

Stir the warmed sugar into the pan over low heat until dissolved, then raise the heat and boil vigorously for 10–15 minutes or until setting point is reached (see page 17).

Remove from the heat and skim the scum from the surface with a slotted spoon. Ladle into warm, clean, dry jars. Cover, seal, and process (see pages 12–13). Leave overnight to set. Store in a cool, dark, dry place.

Serving Suggestion
Use to layer sponge cakes.

Peach Marmalade

I love this marmalade and never tire of eating it. Adjust the cooking time of the orange so that the peel is cooked as tender or as firm as you like.

MAKES ABOUT 3 CUPS

2 large thin-skinned oranges, very thinly sliced
2¼ pounds peaches, peeled, halved, pitted, and chopped
juice of 1 lemon
3⅓ cups warmed sugar (see page 7)

Halve each orange slice, then cut each piece into quarters, reserving the seeds. Tie the seeds in a cheesecloth bag. Put the orange pieces, cheesecloth bag, and ¾ cup water in a small saucepan, cover, and simmer gently for about 40 minutes or until the orange peel is tender.

Pour the contents of the pan into a large saucepan and tie the loose end of the cheesecloth bag string onto the pan handle so that the bag is suspended in the mixture. Add the peaches and lemon juice and simmer until tender. Lift out the cheesecloth bag with a slotted spoon and press it firmly with the back of a metal spoon so that the juices run back into the pan. Discard the bag.

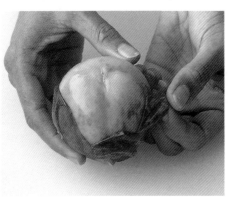

Peeling peaches: Pour boiling water over the peaches and leave for 10–30 seconds, depending on their ripeness, before peeling.

Over low heat, stir in the warmed sugar until it has dissolved. Raise the heat and boil vigorously for 10–15 minutes or until setting point is reached (see page 17). Ladle into warm, clean, dry jars. Cover, seal, and process (see pages 12–13). Leave overnight to set. Store in a cool, dark, dry place.

Serving Suggestion
Serve this lovely marmalade with a Continental breakfast of warmed croissants and brioches or as a filling for sponge cakes.

Spiced Peaches

This particular blend of spices gives the peaches a slightly exotic taste.

MAKES 5 CUPS

4½ cups sugar
2½ cups white wine vinegar
2 cinnamon sticks
12 black peppercorns
4 cardamom pods, crushed
1 teaspoon whole cloves
2 star anise
4 pounds peaches, peeled, halved, and pitted

In a large saucepan, gently heat the sugar in the vinegar with the spices, stirring, until the sugar has dissolved. Raise the heat and boil the mixture for 2–2½ minutes. Add the peach halves and simmer for 4–5 minutes or until they are tender.

Using a slotted spoon, transfer the peaches to a clean, warm, dry jar. Reduce the liquid slightly by boiling it for 2–3 minutes, then pour over the peaches. Rotate the jar to expel any air bubbles, then cover, seal, and process (see pages 12–13). Store the peaches in a cool, dark, dry place for at least 2 months before eating.

Serving Suggestion
Eat with turkey, duck, pork, or cold ham.

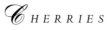
Black Cherry Jam with Kirsch

The cherries for this jam must be acidic cherries, not just any variety. But even sour cherries are very low in pectin, so I add pectin extract to encourage a good set and keep the cooking time down.

MAKES ABOUT 4 CUPS

2 pounds black sour cherries, pitted
commercial liquid pectin or ⅔ cup pectin
** extract (see page 7)**
5 cups sugar
1 tablespoon kirsch

In a large saucepan, gently heat the cherries, pectin extract and sugar until the sugar has dissolved, then simmer until the cherries are just tender (if using commercial pectin, follow the manufacturer's directions).

Raise the heat and bring to a boil, then boil vigorously for about 4 minutes or until setting point is reached (see page 17).

Remove the pan from the heat and skim any scum that has formed on the surface with a slotted spoon. Stir the kirsch into the jam, then ladle it into warm, clean, dry jars. Cover, seal, and process (see pages 12–13). Leave the jam overnight to set. Store in a cool, dark, dry place.

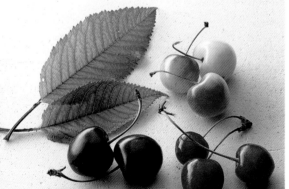

Serving Suggestion
Serve as a topping for a cheesecake; in Black Forest gâteau; with whipped cream in a chocolate roulade; with roast or broiled duck or roast turkey.

Spiced Cherries

The inspiration for these cherries came from the Italian preserve *amarena fabbri*, available only from a few specialty shops.

MAKES ABOUT 3⅓ CUPS

¼-ounce piece of fresh ginger
2¼ cups granulated sugar
1-inch piece cinnamon stick
3 whole cloves
1¼ cups red wine vinegar
2 pounds sour cherries, pitted

Bruise the ginger with the flat side of a large knife on a chopping board.

In a large saucepan, gently heat the sugar, ginger, and other spices in the vinegar until the sugar has dissolved. Add the cherries and simmer gently until they are tender.

Using a slotted spoon, transfer the cherries to a nonmetallic sieve placed over a bowl. Boil the vinegar until reduced to a thick syrup, adding the juices collected in the bowl. Scoop out the spices with a slotted spoon.

Return the cherries to the syrup and bring to a boil, then pour into warm, clean, dry jars. Cover with acid-proof lids, seal, and process (see pages 12–13). Store the cherries in a cool, dark, dry place for at least 2 weeks before using.

Serving Suggestion
Extremely good with roast game, especially venison and duck, or added to casseroles.

Left (clockwise from top): Pale Duke, Morello, and black cherries.

Savory Cherry Spread

On a recent visit to a nearby country market, I found a small stall selling a variety of assorted preserves. Everything was sparkling, and all the products looked delicious, so I bought a selection. The preserves were so good, in fact, that I went back to the same stall and managed to get the recipe for this spread.

MAKES ABOUT 3 CUPS

2 pounds sour cherries, pitted
1⅓ cups plump raisins
2 teaspoons apple pie spice
1¼ cups cider vinegar
1¼ cups light brown sugar, warmed
** (see page 7)**
⅓ cup clear honey

Put the cherries, raisins, apple pie spice, and vinegar into a pan and bring to a boil, then simmer until the cherries are tender. Press the mixture through a nonmetallic sieve with a wooden spoon, making sure you push as much through the sieve as possible.

Return the mixture to the rinsed pan and, over low heat, stir in the sugar and honey until the sugar has dissolved. Raise the heat and bring to a boil, then lower the heat again and boil, stirring as necessary, for 45–55 minutes or until the mixture is so thick that the spoon leaves a clear line when drawn through it.

Spoon the spread into small warm, clean, dry jars or lightly oiled decorative molds. Cover, seal, and process (see pages 12–13). Store in a cool, dark, dry place for 2–3 months before eating.

Serving Suggestion
Serve this spread with game, lamb, cold ham, or bacon.

$\mathcal{C}$HERRIES

Cherries in Almond Syrup

Morello and Montmorency cherries are traditional acidic varieties, whereas Dukes are sweet-sour, so use the ones that will produce the flavor you most enjoy.

Adding the cracked cherry pits when cooking the cherries imparts an almond flavor. You can boost it further by pouring some almond liqueur into the bottles.

MAKES ABOUT 3½ QUARTS

3 pounds Morello, Montmorency, or Duke cherries (see above)
3⅛ cups sugar

Remove the pits from the cherries, reserving a small handful of the pits. Tie them in a square of cheesecloth and hit firmly with a rolling pin to crack them.

In a large saucepan, gently heat the sugar in 7½ cups water, stirring, until the sugar has dissolved. Add the cheesecloth bag (tying the loose end of the string to the pan handle so that the bag is suspended in the mixture), raise the heat, and boil for 5 minutes.

Add the cherries and cook over moderate heat for about 5 minutes. Using a slotted spoon, carefully transfer the cherries to warm, clean, dry jars.

Boil the syrup for another 5 minutes or until slightly reduced, then discard the cheesecloth bag. Pour the syrup over the cherries, making sure they are completely covered. Cover and seal the jars (see pages 12–13). Process in a boiling water bath (see page 13) for 10 minutes. Remove the jars from the heat, tighten the lids, then leave to cool and test the seals. Store in a cool, dark, dry place for 2–3 days before eating.

Serving Suggestion
The cherries can be used in almost any sweet recipe calling for cherries – in pie, crêpe, and sweet omelet fillings; stirred into plain cake batters; added to strudel fillings; spooned over ice cream; or included in ice cream sundaes.

Variation: *Peaches in Almond Syrup*
Peel, halve, and pit the peaches. Follow the recipe above. Makes 3½ quarts.

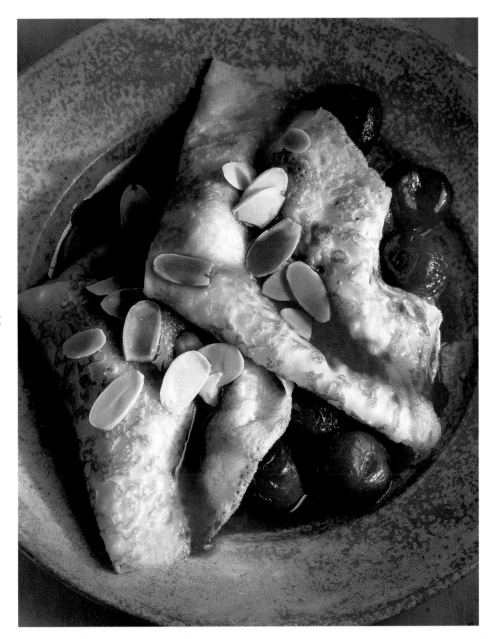

Above: Cherries in Almond Syrup makes a quick and delectable filling for a light dessert of almond crêpes.

Damson Plum Jam

Cinnamon and orange highlight the spicy flavor of damson plums. There is no need to pit the fruit before cooking, or to worry about hurrying when removing the pits after the jam has been cooked. A 10–15 minute delay is needed anyway before putting it into jars; otherwise the fruit skins will float to the surface of the jam in the jars.

MAKES ABOUT 5⅓ CUPS

grated zest and juice of 3 oranges
2½ pounds damson plums
1½ teaspoons ground cinnamon
5¾ cups warmed sugar (see page 7)

Add water to the orange juice to make 1¼ cups, then put in a large saucepan with the plums, cinnamon, and orange zest. Cook gently in the liquid for about 40 minutes or until the fruit is very tender and the liquid well reduced.

Over low heat, stir in the warmed sugar until it has dissolved. Raise the heat and boil for about 10 minutes, stirring occasionally, until setting point is reached (see page 17).

Remove from the heat and take out the plum pits with a slotted spoon. Put the pits in a nonmetallic sieve over the pan to drain for about 15 minutes. Skim the surface with a slotted spoon. Stir the jam, then ladle it into warm, clean, dry jars. Cover, seal, and process (see pages 12–13). Leave overnight to set. Store in a cool, dark, dry place.

Variations: *Plum Jam*
Use 3 pounds plums, 1¼ cups water, and 7 cups sugar. Halve and pit the plums, reserving about 14 of the pits. Crack the reserved plum pits (see page 108), remove the kernels, and add them to the pan with the water and plums (the kernels add a complementary almond flavor). Simmer for 20–30 minutes or until the plum skins are soft. Proceed with the recipe above. Makes about 5⅔ cups.

Instead of adding the kernels, you could add orange zest and juice, as in the recipe for Damson Plum Jam.
Greengage Plum Jam
Use 3 pounds greengage plums, 1¼ cups water, and 7 cups sugar. Cook the whole plums in the water until very soft, then proceed with the recipe above. Makes about 6⅔ cups.

Damson Plum Spread

This is a dark and richly flavored spread.

MAKES ABOUT 4 CUPS

3 pounds damson plums
warmed sugar (see page 7)

Just cover the plums with water and simmer for 15-20 minutes or until the fruit is very soft and no surplus water is visible. Scoop out the pits as they rise to the surface, using a slotted spoon.

Press the plums through a nonmetallic sieve and measure the purée. Return the purée to the pan with 1¾ cups sugar for every 2½ cups purée. Heat gently, stirring, until the sugar has dissolved, then boil gently, stirring frequently, for 45–55 minutes or until the mixture is so thick that when the wooden spoon is drawn across the bottom of the pan, a clean line is left.

Spoon the spread into warm, clean, dry jars or lightly oiled small dishes or molds. Cover, seal, and process (see pages 12–13). Store the spread in a cool, dark, dry place for 2–3 months before eating.

Serving Suggestion
Serve with aged Cheddar cheese or cream cheese; with firm white bread and unsalted butter; with warm gingerbread; or as a condiment for roast lamb, duck, or game.

Plum Gin

Plums are used to make a number of different alcoholic drinks, which differ in character according to the variety of plum used. The best known alcoholic plum drink is *slivovitz*, a plum brandy made by distilling the fruit. This is illegal to make at home, of course, without a special licence, so I make my own plum alcoholic drink by steeping plums in gin.

MAKES ABOUT 3½ CUPS

1 pound dark plums
7 tablespoons sugar
a few blanched almonds, lightly crushed
1 750ml bottle of gin

Prick each plum all over with a large embroidery needle or round wooden toothpick, then layer with the sugar and almonds in a clean jar. Pour the gin over the plums to cover completely.

Close the jar tightly, shake it well, and leave in a cool, dark, dry place for at least 3 months, shaking the jar occasionally.

Strain the gin through a nonmetallic funnel lined with cheesecloth into clean, dry bottles. Seal the bottles (see pages 12–13). Store in a cool, dark, dry place.

Serving Suggestion
As well as a warming drink, plum gin can be used to liven up meat and game casseroles and sauces (see page 105).

Variations: *Plum Vodka*
Use vodka in place of gin. Plum vodka has a cleaner, fruitier taste than plum gin. Makes about 3½ cups.
Damson Plum Brandy
Use about 1 pound damson plums and brandy instead of the plums and gin and omit the almonds. Follow the main recipe. Makes about 3½ cups.

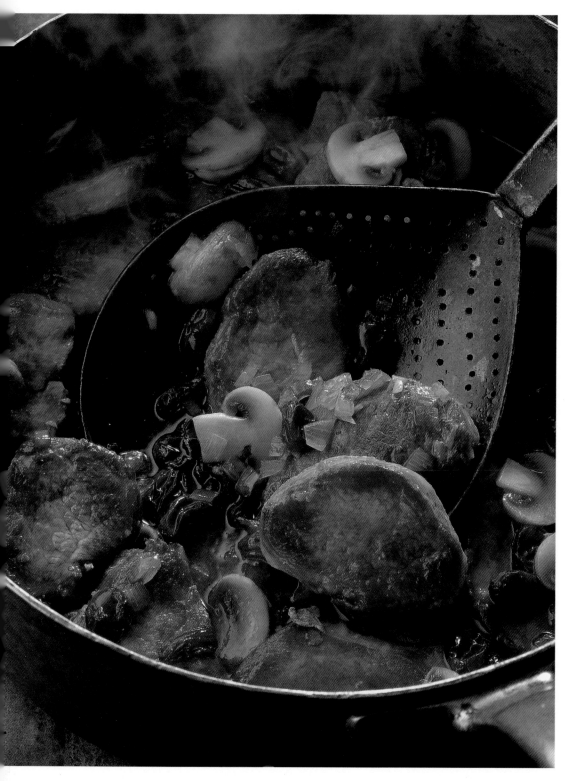

Pork with Plum Gin Sauce

Plum gin cuts through the creamy sauce in this recipe and enhances the flavor of the sliced pork.

SERVES 6

2 tablespoons unsalted butter
2 tablespoons olive oil
2 pounds pork tenderloin, cut into ½-inch thick slices
1 shallot, chopped
4½ ounces button mushrooms, sliced
¼ cup Plum Gin (see page 104)
1¼ cups beef stock
½ cup plump raisins
⅔ cup crème fraîche or heavy cream
table salt and freshly ground black pepper

Heat the butter and oil in a heavy skillet and brown the pork on both sides in batches. Remove with a slotted spoon and drain on paper towels.

Add the shallot and mushrooms to the skillet and cook gently until softened but not colored. Stir in the plum gin to dislodge the pan juices, then bring to a boil. Add the stock and raisins and return to a simmer, then add the pork, cover tightly, and cook gently for 10–15 minutes or until tender.

Transfer the pork to a warm serving dish, cover, and keep warm. Boil the sauce vigorously until slightly reduced, then stir in the crème fraîche or heavy cream and boil vigorously again until slightly syrupy. Season with salt and pepper and pour over the pork while still hot.

Left: Plum Gin combined with gently cooked shallots and raisins makes a richly flavored sauce for this memorable pork dish.

Plum and Red Onion Confit

Szechuan peppercorns give a wonderful spicy-woody flavor to this confit. I give the onions just a short cooking on their own so that they retain some texture in the end.

MAKES ABOUT 2⅓ CUPS

1 pound red onions, chopped
2 tablespoons olive oil
1 tablespoon Szechuan peppercorns
1½ pounds red plums, halved and pitted
1¼ cups red wine vinegar
sea salt
10–14 tablespoons brown sugar, warmed (see page 7)

Gently cook the onions in the oil in a large saucepan until they are as soft as you like.

Meanwhile, heat the peppercorns in a dry heavy skillet until fragrant, moving them gently around the pan to prevent them from burning. Remove from the heat then transfer the peppercorns to a mortar and crush finely with a pestle, or grind in a spice grinder or small blender.

Add the plums, peppercorns, vinegar, and salt to the onions and simmer, uncovered, until the plums are tender.

Over low heat, stir in the sugar until dissolved, then simmer until thick.

Spoon the confit into warm, clean, dry jars. Cover, seal, and process (see pages 12–13). Store in a cool, dark, dry place for at least 1 month before eating.

Serving Suggestion
With grilled or broiled good-quality sausages; if the onions still have some bite left after the cooking, the relish can accompany mackerel.

Right: Plum and Red Onion Confit adds spice to a dish of finest-quality broiled sausages and a light purée of buttered potatoes.

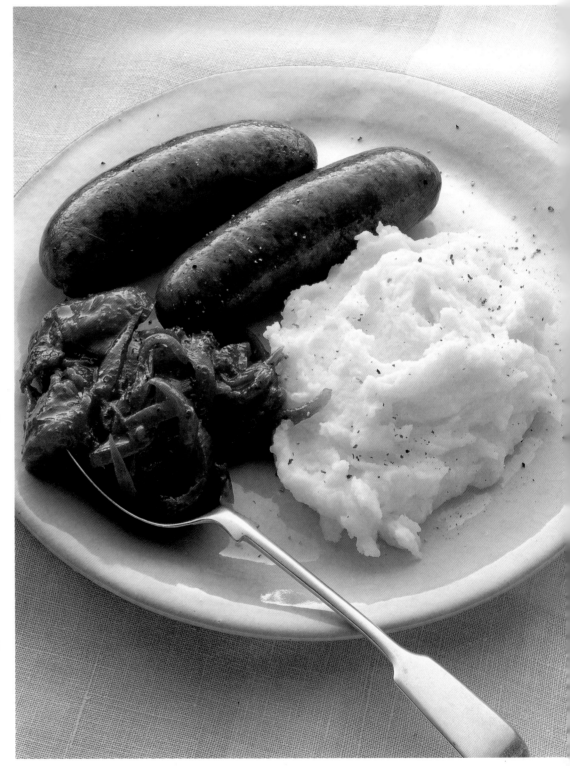

Plum Jelly

MAKES 3²/₃–4 CUPS

commercial liquid pectin or 1 cup pectin extract (see page 7)
3 pounds plums, halved and pitted
7 cups warmed sugar (see page 7)

Put the pectin extract, plums, and 3½ cups water into a saucepan and bring to a boil, then simmer for 20–30 minutes or until the plums are tender (if using commercial pectin, follow the manfacturer's directions).

Pour the contents of the pan into a scalded jelly bag suspended over a large nonmetallic bowl and leave to strain, undisturbed, in a cool place for 8–12 hours.

Measure the strained juice – there should be about 1½ quarts. If there is not enough, make up the quantity with water; if there is too much, add extra sugar in equal quantity to the extra juice. Pour into the rinsed pan, add the remaining sugar, and heat gently, stirring, until the sugar has dissolved. Raise the heat and boil for 1 minute or until the setting point is reached (see page 17).

Remove from the heat and skim any scum from the surface. Immediately ladle into warm, clean, dry jars. Cover, seal, and process (see pages 12–13). Leave overnight to set. Store in a cool, dark, dry place.

Plum Sauce

MAKES ABOUT 3 CUPS

½ cinnamon stick
4 whole cloves
2 star anise
5 coriander seeds, lightly crushed
²/₃ cup cider vinegar
1 pound plums, pitted and chopped
1 shallot, chopped
5 tablespoons each port and Madeira
juice each of ½ large lemon, ½ orange, and ½ lime

pinch of five-spice powder
1 tablespoon red currant jelly
⅓ cup warmed demerara or raw sugar (see page 7)

Tie the cinnamon stick, cloves, star anise, and coriander seeds in a cheesecloth bag. Put the remaining ingredients except the sugar into a large saucepan. Tie the loose string of the cheesecloth bag onto the pan handle so that the bag is suspended in the mixture. Bring to a boil, then simmer gently for about 45 minutes, stirring occasionally. Stir in the warmed sugar until it has dissolved, then continue to simmer gently for another 45 minutes.

Discard the cheesecloth bag, pour the sauce into a blender, and purée. Pour the sauce into warm, clean, dry bottles. Cover and seal (see pages 12–13). Store in a cool, dark, dry place for 1 month before using.

Spiced Plums

MAKES ABOUT 6 CUPS

2 pounds 14 ounces purple plums
3⅓ cups sugar
½ ounce fresh ginger, grated
½ teaspoon whole cloves

½ teaspoon ground coriander seeds
½ teaspoon ground allspice
¼ cinnamon stick
2 cups red wine vinegar

Prick the fruit all over with a round wooden toothpick and put in a pan large enough so that the fruit is no more than 2 layers deep.

In another pan, gently heat the sugar and spices in the vinegar, stirring, until the sugar has dissolved. Raise the heat and bring to a boil, then simmer for 5 minutes.

Pour the spiced vinegar into the fruit pan and heat until boiling. Remove from the heat, cover, and leave for about 8 hours.

Strain off the liquid through a nonmetallic sieve and reserve. Using a slotted spoon, pack the fruit into warm, clean, dry jars. Boil the liquid vigorously until reduced by one-third, then pour it into the jars to cover the fruit. Rotate the jars to dispel any air bubbles, then immediately cover the jars with acid-proof lids, seal, and process (see pages 12–13). Store the plums in a cool, dark, dry place for 1 month before using.

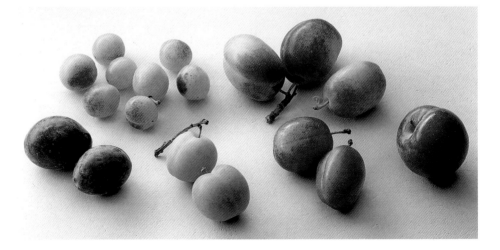

Below (clockwise from bottom left): Damson, Mirabelle, Victoria, red and greengage plums.

Autumn Chutney

Bringing together the fruits of the orchard – apples, pears, and plums – this chutney can be made in the fall and put by for serving with cheeses in later months.

MAKES ABOUT 6 CUPS

1 pound Victoria plums, pitted (see below) and very finely chopped
1 pound each pears and cooking apples, cored and cut into chunks without peeling
1⅓ cups raisins
1½ cups onions, very finely chopped
finely grated peel and juice of 1 orange
2½ cups cider vinegar
1¾ cups warmed light brown sugar (see page 7)
¼ teaspoon each ground cinnamon, ground ginger, and ground cloves

Put the fruit, raisins, onions, orange zest and juice, and vinegar in a large saucepan and bring to a boil, then simmer for about 45 minutes, stirring occasionally, until the fruit is tender.

Over low heat, stir in the warmed sugar and the spices until the sugar has dissolved. Then simmer, stirring occasionally, until the chutney is thick and there is no free liquid.

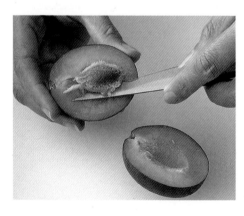

Removing pits from plums: Cut the fruit in half, following the natural indentation, then cut out the pit with a knife.

Ladle the chutney into warm, clean, dry jars, taking care not to trap any air bubbles. Cover the jars with acid-proof lids, seal, and process (see pages 12–13). Store the chutney in a cool, dark, dry place for at least 2 months before eating.

Fresh Date and Orange Chutney

The date palm was the tree of life in the Garden of Eden. There is even an Arab belief that when Allah created the world, he formed the date palm not from common clay but from the material remaining after he had built Adam.

MAKES ABOUT 4 CUPS

1 pound oranges
1½ pounds fresh dates, pitted and finely chopped
1 pound onions, finely chopped
3 garlic cloves, finely chopped
4 ounces dried apricot halves, chopped
⅔ cup raisins
3¾ cups light brown sugar
good pinch of cayenne pepper
2 tablespoons sea salt
10 cups white wine vinegar

Grate the zest from the oranges, then, working over a bowl, peel off and discard the white pith from the fruit. Chop the flesh into a large saucepan so as not to waste any juice; discard the seeds. Add any juice collected in the bowl, half of the zest, and all the remaining ingredients to the pan and heat gently, stirring, until the sugar has dissolved. Raise the heat and bring to a boil, then simmer gently for about 1 hour, stirring occasionally, until thick and there is no free liquid. Stir in the remaining orange zest.

Spoon into warm, clean, dry jars; do not trap any air bubbles. Cover, seal, and process (see pages 12–13). Store the chutney in a cool, dark, dry place for at least 4–6 weeks before eating.

Fresh Date and Pineapple Chutney

The original version I have of this recipe comes from before the Second World War, so it called for dried dates and canned pineapple. That chutney was quite good but not particularly special. If you use fresh dates and pineapples, which are now readily available, the chutney is transformed.

MAKES ABOUT 6 CUPS

8 ounces onions, chopped
1 pineapple, about 3 pounds, peeled, cored, and cut into small pieces
1 pound cooking apples, peeled, cored, and chopped
1 teaspoon ground cinnamon
scant 2 cups cider vinegar
8 ounces fresh dates, pitted and coarsely chopped
1¼ cups warmed light brown sugar (see page 7)

Gently simmer the onions, pineapple, apples, cinnamon, and vinegar for 30–40 minutes or until the fruit is soft.

Stir in the dates and warmed sugar until it has dissolved, then bring slowly to a boil and boil gently for 20–25 minutes, stirring frequently, until the fruit is well coated in thick syrup.

Ladle the chutney into warm, clean, dry jars, making sure that you do not trap any air bubbles. Cover the jars with acid-proof lids, seal, and process (see pages 12–13). Store in a cool, dark, dry place for 2 months before eating.

Mango Butter

Shortly before the butter is ready, taste it to see if the cardamom flavor is strong enough; if it is not, toast and crush a few more seeds to stir in. Alternatively, have some more prepared just in case.

MAKES ABOUT 3⅓ CUPS

½ teaspoon cardamom seeds
2 pounds fresh mango pulp
½ cup lemon juice
½ cup orange juice
2 cups warmed sugar (see page 7)

Heat the cardamom seeds in a dry small heavy skillet until fragrant, moving them gently around the pan to prevent them from burning. Remove the seeds from the pan and crush them using a mortar and pestle or a small blender; set aside.

Cut the mango flesh from the pits, then chop it and put in a large saucepan with the lemon and orange juices. Bring to a boil, then simmer, stirring occasionally, until the mangoes are soft and there is no free liquid.

Press the mangoes through a fine nonmetallic sieve with a wooden spoon and return to the rinsed pan. Over low heat, stir in the warmed sugar and the cardamom seeds and heat gently, stirring, until the sugar has dissolved. Boil, stirring occasionally at first, then more frequently, until the mixture has the consistency of sour cream. This should take 30–45 minutes.

Spoon the butter into warm, clean, dry jars. Cover and seal (see pages 12–13). Store in a cool, dark, dry place for a few days before eating.

Serving Suggestion
Serve for breakfast with toasted brioche or warmed croissants.

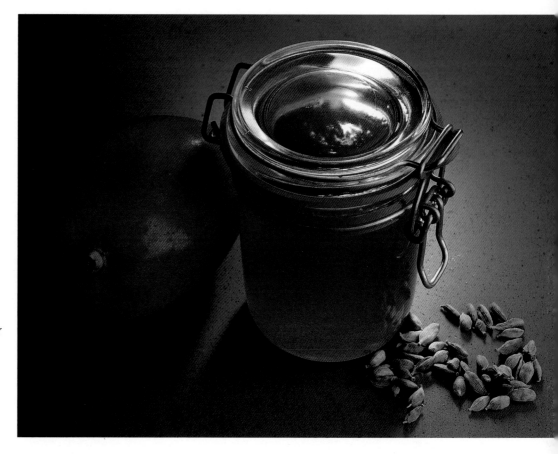

Guava Jelly

Made with slightly underripe fruit, this recipe needs no added pectin.

MAKES ABOUT 2 CUPS

3 pounds guavas, thinly sliced
3 cardamom pods, crushed (optional)
3⅓ cups warmed sugar (see page 7)
juice of 1–2 large lemons, depending on the
  acidity of the guavas

Put the guavas and cardamom pods, if using, into a large saucepan, add water to barely cover, and bring to a boil, then simmer for about 45 minutes or until the fruit is very soft.

Purée the fruit by passing it through a non-metallic sieve or blending it, then pour it into

Above: Mango Butter makes a glamorous and exotically flavored spread.

a scalded jelly bag suspended over a non-metallic bowl and leave in a cool place to strain, undisturbed, for 8–12 hours.

Measure the strained juice and pour it into the pan. Add 2¼ cups sugar for every 2½ cups juice. Add the lemon juice and heat gently, stirring, until the sugar has dissolved. Raise the heat and boil vigorously for 10–15 minutes or until setting point is reached (see page 17).

Remove from the heat and skim the scum from the surface with a slotted spoon. Ladle into warm, clean, dry jars. Cover, seal, and process (see pages 12–13). Leave overnight to set. Store in a cool, dark, dry place.

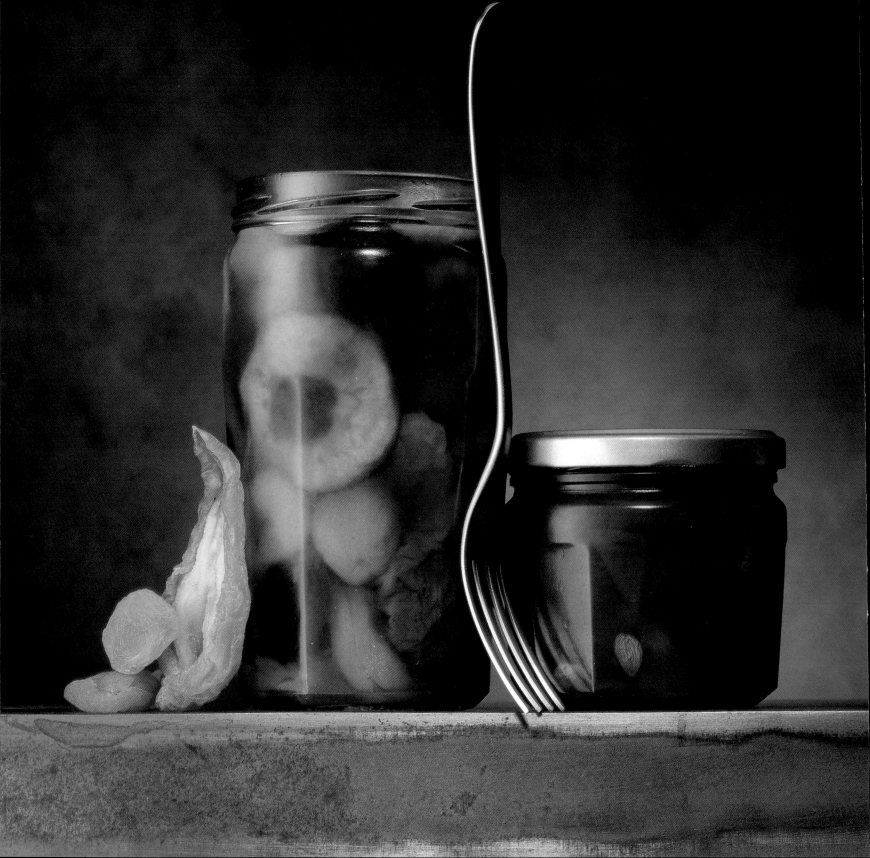

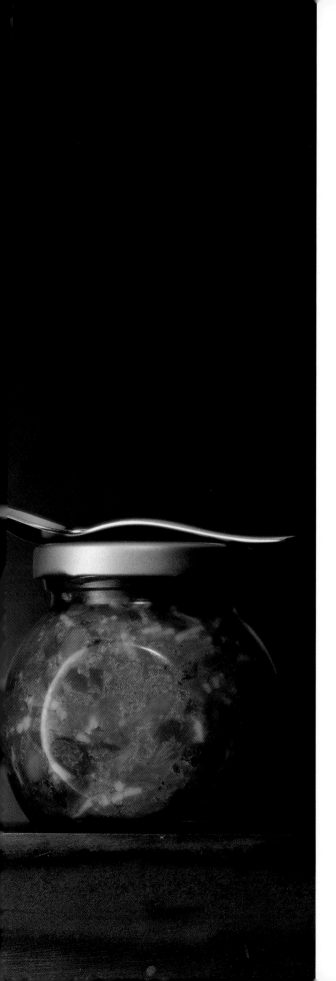

DRIED FRUITS

Shiny black, plump Prunes in Armagnac (see page 114); deep, glowing, amber-colored Dried Apricot and Benedictine Conserve (see page 112); chunky chutneys and spicy piquant pickles can all be prepared inexpensively at any time of the year using a wide variety of dried fruits. An added bonus of using dried fruits is that they rarely need any preparation other than an initial soaking. For the best results, try to find fruit that has been dried naturally in the sun and choose fruits that have not been treated with preservatives such as sulfur dioxide and mineral oils.

Left (from left to right): Spiced Dried Fruits, Dried Apricot and Pear Jam, and Dried Apricot and Orange Mincemeat.

Dried Apricot and Benedictine Conserve

Sufferers from rheumatism have a very good excuse for eating generous amounts of this richly flavored preserve, as Benedictine is reputed to ease such complaints.

MAKES ABOUT 6 CUPS

1 pound dried apricot halves
warmed sugar (see page 7)
grated zest and juice of 1 orange
⅔ cup sliced almonds
¼ cup Benedictine

Put the dried apricot halves and 1¼ quarts water in a nonmetallic bowl and leave them to soak overnight.

Pour the contents of the bowl into a large saucepan and bring to the simmering point, then cover and cook gently for about 45 minutes or until the apricots are very soft.

Purée the apricots by pressing through a nonmetallic sieve or by blending. Measure the purée and return to the pan with 2¼ cups sugar for each 2½ cups purée. Stir in the orange zest and juice and bring to a boil, then boil for about 10 minutes, stirring as necessary, until thick.

Remove from the heat and stir in the almonds and Benedictine. Leave to stand for 10–15 minutes, then stir and ladle into warm, clean, dry jars. Cover, seal, and process (see pages 12–13). Leave overnight to set. Store in a cool, dark, dry place.

Apricot Honey

The dried apricots give this honey a wonderful fruity flavor.

MAKES ABOUT 1 QUART

2 cups dried apricot halves
2 tablespoons lemon juice
½ cup clear honey

Put the apricots in a nonmetallic bowl, pour 3½ cups boiling water over them, and leave to soak for about 4 hours.

Drain the apricots, saving the soaking liquid. Boil the liquid for 15–20 minutes or until reduced to 1¾ cups.

Meanwhile, coarsely chop the apricots. Add to the reduced liquid with the lemon juice and simmer until the fruit is soft.

Pour the contents of the pan into a nonmetallic sieve placed over a nonmetallic bowl. Press firmly with a wooden spoon on the contents of the sieve to force through as much as possible. Return the purée to the pan, then stir in the honey and cook, stirring as necessary, until a clear trail is left on the bottom of the pan when the spoon is drawn through the mixture.

Spoon the honey into warm, clean, dry jars. Cover and seal (see pages 12–13). Store in a cool, dark, dry place.

Dried Apricot, Apple, and Cider Jam

MAKES ABOUT 6⅔ CUPS

1⅓ cups chopped dried apricot halves
2½ cups dry hard cider
2 pounds cooking apples, peeled, cored, and chopped
1½ tablespoons lemon juice
7 cups warmed sugar (see page 7)

Put the apricots into a nonmetallic bowl, add the cider, and leave to soak overnight.

Pour the contents of the bowl into a large saucepan, add the apples, and bring to a boil. Lower the heat and simmer for about 1 hour or until the fruit is soft and pulpy.

Over low heat, stir in the lemon juice and warmed sugar until the sugar has dissolved, then raise the heat and boil vigorously for 10–15 minutes, stirring as necessary, until setting point is reached (see page 17).

Remove from the heat and skim the scum from the surface with a slotted spoon. Ladle into warm, clean, dry jars. Cover, seal, and process (see pages 12–13). Leave overnight to set. Store in a cool, dark, dry place.

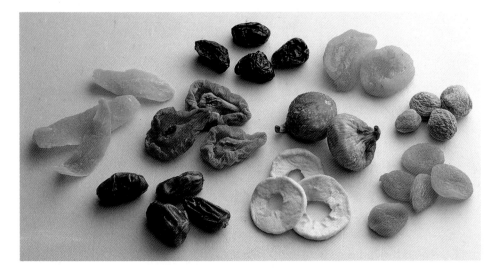

Left (clockwise from top center): Dried prunes, peaches, hunza apricots, apricots, figs, apples, pears, dates, and mango strips.

A PRICOTS

Dried Apricot and Orange Mincemeat

Carrots keep this unusual mincemeat nice and moist, while cardamom adds a subtle complementary note.

MAKES ABOUT 3⅓ CUPS

1⅓ cups chopped dried apricot halves
finely grated zest and juice of 2 large oranges
finely grated zest and juice of 1 lime
1⅓ cups golden raisins
½ cup raisins, chopped
½ cup mixed candied peel
1¼ cups sliced almonds
10 tablespoons dark brown sugar
2 cups carrots, grated
⅔ cup shredded vegetarian or beef suet
seeds from 6 cardamom pods, finely crushed
1½ teaspoons ground cinnamon
½ teaspoon grated nutmeg
¼ cup Cointreau
⅔ cup whiskey

Thoroughly stir all the ingredients together in a large nonmetallic bowl, then cover and leave in a cool place overnight or for at least 8 hours, stirring occasionally.

Pack the mincemeat tightly into clean, dry jars, taking care not to leave any air pockets. Cover, seal, and process (see pages 12–13). Store in a cool, dark, dry place for at least 1 month before eating.

Baked Mincemeat Pudding

SERVES 4

6 tablespoons unsalted butter, softened
6 tablespoons dark brown sugar
2 large eggs, beaten
1 cup self-rising flour
⅔ cup Dried Apricot and Orange Mincemeat
  (see above)
vanilla ice cream for serving

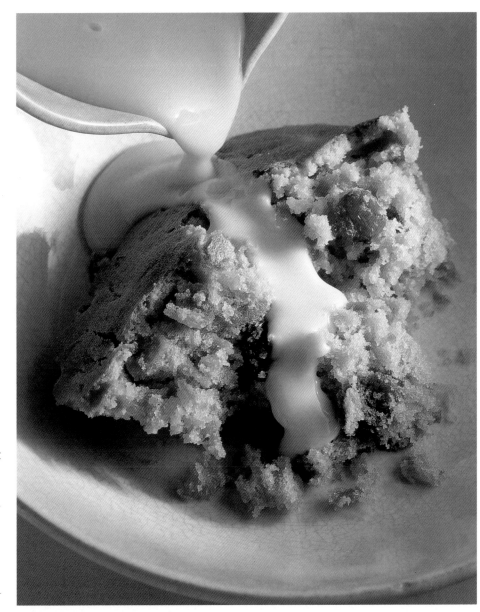

Above: Homemade mincemeat provides the basis for a delicious and speedy Baked Mincemeat Pudding.

Preheat the oven to 325°F and butter an 8-inch shallow, round ovenproof dish.

In a bowl, beat together the butter and sugar until light and fluffy, then gradually beat in the eggs, beating well after each addition. Using a large metal spoon, gently fold in the flour, followed by the mincemeat. Spoon the mixture into the dish and bake for

10 minutes. Lower the oven temperature to 300°F and bake for another 40–45 minutes or until a knife inserted in the center comes out clean. Serve this sensational pudding hot with vanilla ice cream.

Dried Apricot and Pear Jam

Dried apricots and pears make a well-flavored jam, and they really come into their own for making jam in the winter when fresh fruit is scarce and expensive.

MAKES ABOUT 6⅓ CUPS

1½ cups dried apricots
1 pound dried pears
1 vanilla bean
1 cinnamon stick
grated zest and juice of 2 lemons
warmed sugar (see page 7)

Soak the apricots for several hours in 1¼ quarts water. Drain the apricots, reserving the liquid.

Put the pears, vanilla bean, cinnamon stick, lemon zest and juice, 3½ cups water, and the reserved liquid in a large saucepan, bring to a boil, then reduce the heat and simmer for about 10 minutes, stirring occasionally, until the pears are tender.

Over low heat, stir the warmed sugar and apricots into the pan until the sugar has dissolved. Raise the heat and boil for about 20 minutes, stirring frequently, until setting point is reached (see page 17). Remove the vanilla bean and cinnamon stick.

Remove from the heat and leave for about 15 minutes, then ladle into warm, clean, dry jars. Cover, seal, and process (see pages 12–13). Leave overnight to set. Store in a cool, dark, dry place.

Variation: *Dried Apricot and Hazelnut Jam*
Soak 1 pound dried apricot halves in 7½ cups water overnight, then cook in the water and juice of 1 large lemon until soft. Over low heat, stir in 7 cups sugar until dissolved. Just before spooning the jam into jars, add ½ cup toasted and chopped hazelnuts. Makes about 6⅔ cups.

Dried Peach and Chestnut Chutney

I have used cooked chestnuts for this chunky, nutty chutney, but chopped walnuts, almonds, or hazelnuts can easily be substituted.

MAKES ABOUT 5⅓ CUPS

1 pound dried peaches
3 cups chopped onions
finely grated zest and juice of 2 large oranges
1⅓ cups raisins
1 garlic clove, chopped
1 teaspoon dry English mustard
½ teaspoon ground allspice
2¼ cups light brown sugar
3½ cups cider vinegar
1 cup cooked chestnuts, quartered

Place the peaches in a nonmetallic bowl and pour in cold water just to cover them.

The next day, drain the peaches, reserving the liquid, then chop them. Pour the liquid into a large saucepan and boil until well reduced. Stir in the remaining ingredients, except the chestnuts and bring to a boil. Lower the heat and simmer for 1 hour, stirring frequently, until the mixture is thick and jamlike and there is no free liquid.

Remove from the heat and stir in the nuts, then ladle the chutney into warm, clean, dry jars, pressing down to expel any air. Cover with acid-proof lids, seal, and process (see pages 12–13). Store in a cool, dark, dry place for 1 month before eating.

Prunes in Armagnac

As well as being a good way of making the most of good-quality prunes, this recipe is excellent for improving inferior ones. Dry the orange peel in an oven set to the lowest temperature. When choosing a jar to pack the prunes in, don't forget that they will swell during storage.

MAKES ABOUT 1 QUART

1 pound plump prunes
1¾ cups freshly made hot, fragrant tea, such as orange pekoe or Earl Grey
1 strip dried orange peel
1 cup Armagnac brandy
10 tablespoons brown sugar

Place the prunes and tea in a large saucepan and bring to a boil, then simmer for 3 minutes and remove from the heat. Strain off and reserve the liquid.

Pack the prunes into a clean, dry jar, inserting the orange peel at the same time. Pour in the Armagnac.

Return the reserved liquid to the pan, add the sugar, and heat gently, stirring, until it has dissolved. Raise the heat and bring to a boil, then simmer until syrupy. Pour into the jar so that the prunes are well covered.

Rotate the jar to expel any air, then cover tightly. Leave in a cool, dark, dry place for up to 2 months, shaking the jar occasionally, before eating.

Serving Suggestion
Serve with roast pork or duck; dilute the juice slightly and use to deglaze a pan after frying pork steaks, then serve along with some of the prunes; use as a simple dessert accompanied by ice cream; eat both chilled prunes and juice with a crisp almond cookie; add to fruit salads.

Variation: *Prunes in Rum*
Replace the Armagnac with rum and proceed as above. Makes about 1 quart.

PRUNES

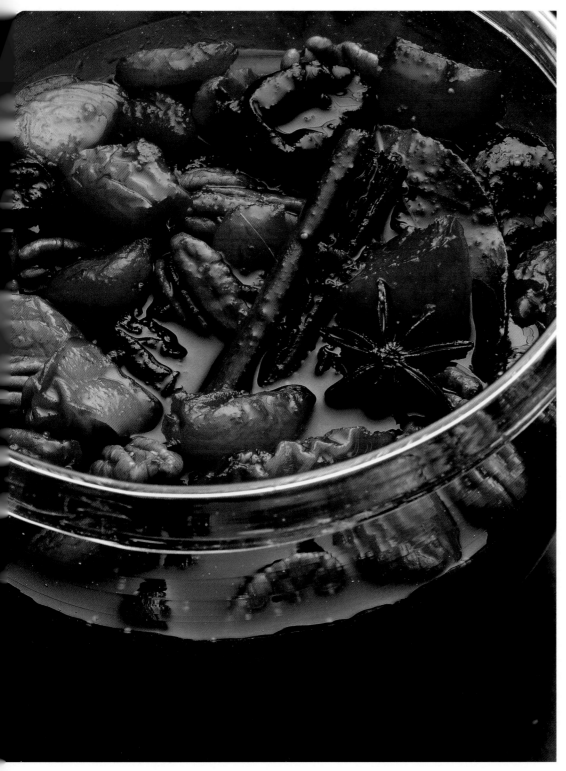

Prune, Dried Fruit, and Pecan Compote

A few jars of this compote will come in handy during the winter for quick or impromptu desserts or will add a taste of luxury to plain ones. If you want a less spicy mixture, put all the spices in a cheesecloth bag and discard after the soaking.

MAKES ABOUT 2 QUARTS

3 cups red wine
1 bay leaf
4 whole cloves
1 cinnamon stick
2 star anise
1 vanilla bean
½ teaspoon coriander seeds
5 black peppercorns
12 ounces prunes, pitted
1½ pounds mixed dried apricot halves, peaches, pears, and figs, coarsely chopped
½ cup pecans
1¼ cups sugar
¼ cup brandy

Simmer the wine with the spices for 30 minutes. Pour over the fruit in a nonmetallic bowl and leave to soak overnight.

Using a slotted spoon, pack the fruit into clean, dry, heatproof jars with the spices, if retaining. Put the nuts in among the fruit.

Pour the wine into a large saucepan, add the sugar, and heat gently, stirring, until the sugar has dissolved. Raise the heat and boil until syrupy.

Remove from the heat, add the brandy, and ladle into the jars. Rotate the jars to expel any air. Cover, seal, and process (see pages 12–13). Store in a cool, dark, dry place for 3–4 weeks before eating.

Left: Prune, Dried Fruit, and Pecan Compote, a deliciously nutty and textured preserve.

115

Prune and Raisin Conserve

MAKES ABOUT 4⅔ CUPS

1¼ pounds prunes, halved and pitted
2 cups raisins
⅔ cup chopped dried figs or pitted dates
2¼ cups freshly made hot Earl Grey tea
finely grated zest and juice of 1 orange
juice of 1 lemon
2 whole cloves
1¼ cups dark brown sugar, warmed
  (see page 7)
½ cup walnut halves
¼ cup kirsch or dark rum

Put all the dried fruits into a bowl, pour in the tea, cover, and leave overnight.

Pour the contents of the bowl into a large saucepan, add the remaining ingredients except the nuts and kirsch or rum, and heat gently, stirring, until the sugar has dissolved. Raise the heat and bring to a boil, then simmer for about 12 minutes, stirring, until a light setting point is reached (see page 17).

Remove the pan from the heat, add the nuts and kirsch or rum, and ladle into warm, clean, dry jars. Cover, seal, and process (see pages 12–13). Store in a cool, dark, dry place for several days before eating.

Spiced Prunes

MAKES ABOUT 3 CUPS

1 pound plump prunes
2 cups freshly made hot Earl Grey tea
10 tablespoons sugar
1 teaspoon whole cloves
8 allspice berries
1 blade of mace
1-inch piece cinnamon stick
⅔ cup white wine vinegar
few short strips of orange zest

Soak the prunes in the tea in a covered nonmetallic bowl overnight.

The next day, place the sugar, spices, and vinegar in a pan and heat gently, stirring, until the sugar has dissolved, then raise the heat and boil for 5 minutes. Add the prunes and their soaking liquid, cover, and simmer gently for about 20 minutes or until tender.

Using a slotted spoon, pack the prunes firmly into a warm, clean, dry jar, pushing some short strips of orange zest among the fruit. Bring the liquid to a boil, then pour it over the prunes. Rotate the jar to dispel air bubbles. Cover with acid-proof lids, seal, and process (see pages 12–13). Store in a cool, dark, dry place for 1 month before eating.

Serving Suggestion
Serve with ham, pork, duck, or squab; braise with red cabbage; use a little of the juice to deglaze the juices of roast meats.

Dried Fruit Chutney

You can either chop the dried fruits coarsely for a chunky chutney or finely for a smoother one.

MAKES ABOUT 6⅔ CUPS

8 ounces dried peaches, chopped
8 ounces dried apricots, chopped
8 ounces dried pears, chopped
2½ cups white wine vinegar
1 pound cooking apples, peeled, cored,
  and chopped
1½ cups finely chopped onions
2 garlic cloves, finely chopped
⅔ cup raisins
½ teaspoon ground coriander
½ teaspoon ground cloves
1 teaspoon dry English mustard
good pinch of cayenne pepper
1 teaspoon sea salt
3⅓ cups light brown sugar, warmed
  (see page 7)

Leave the dried peaches, apricots, and pears to soak in the vinegar in a nonmetallic bowl overnight.

The next day, pour the contents of the bowl into a large saucepan and bring to a boil, then add the remaining ingredients except the sugar and simmer for 30 minutes or until all the fruits are tender.

Over low heat, stir in the warmed sugar until it has dissolved. Raise the heat and boil, stirring frequently, for 15–20 minutes or until the ingredients are tender and the chutney is thick and there is no free liquid.

Spoon into warm, clean, dry jars, taking care not to leave any air bubbles. Cover with acid-proof lids, seal, and process (see pages 12–13). Store in a cool, dark, dry place for 2 months before eating.

Spiced Dried Fruits

These spiced dried fruits are sweet enough to serve on their own for dessert (you can add a little sugar if they are not sweet enough for your taste). They can also be served with meats or added to pork, lamb, or pheasant casseroles (see page 117).

MAKES ABOUT 4 CUPS

2 pounds mixed dried fruit, such as prunes,
  apple rings, pears, peaches, and apricots
2-inch piece of fresh ginger, grated
2 teaspoons each allspice berries and whole
  cloves
1 cinnamon stick
pared zest of 1 lemon
1⅔ cups cider vinegar
2 cups sugar

Put all the dried fruit in a nonmetallic bowl, cover it with water, cover the bowl, and leave to soak overnight.

Place the ginger, allspice, cloves, cinnamon stick, lemon zest, and vinegar in a pan and bring to a boil, then simmer for 10 minutes. Leave to cool.

Meanwhile, pour the dried fruits and their soaking liquid into a pan and simmer gently, covered, until tender.

Strain the vinegar through a nonmetallic sieve lined with cheesecloth, discarding the spices and zest, and return it to the pan. Add the sugar and heat gently, stirring, until it has dissolved. Raise the heat and bring to a boil, then simmer for 7–10 minutes or until the vinegar is syrupy.

Drain the fruits. Pack into warm, clean, dry jars. Pour in the hot vinegar to cover. Rotate the jars to expel any air. Cover with acid-proof lids, seal, and process (see pages 12–13). Store in a cool, dark, dry place for at least 1 month before eating.

Braised Lamb with Spiced Dried Fruits

This can be cooked one day in advance up to when the dried fruits are added. The next day, 30 minutes before serving, bring the casserole slowly to a boil, cover, and simmer for about 20 minutes, adding the fruits halfway through.

SERVES 4

1½ pounds boned leg of lamb, cubed
1½ tablespoons mild olive oil
1 onion, finely chopped
1 garlic clove, finely chopped
2 teaspoons all-purpose flour
1 cinnamon stick
1 teaspoon ground allspice
2 cups chicken stock
finely grated zest and juice of 1 orange
finely grated zest and juice of ½ lemon
7 tablespoons spiced vinegar from Spiced
   Dried Fruits (see page 116)
about 1 tablespoon clear honey
pinch of cayenne pepper
salt and freshly ground black pepper
about 10 pieces of Spiced Dried Fruit,
   halved if large

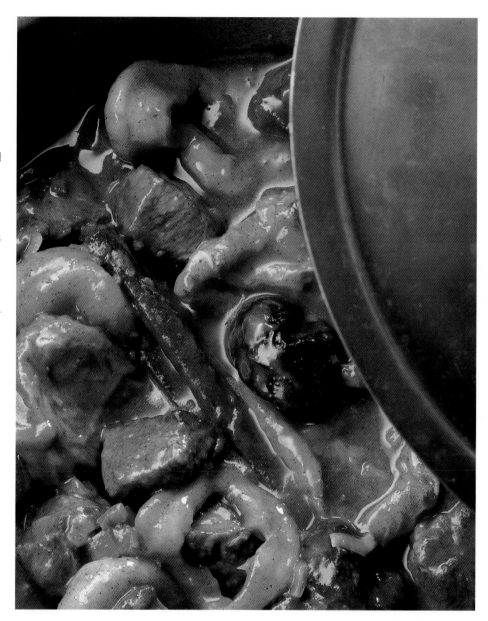

Preheat the oven to 325°F.

Brown the lamb in batches in the oil in a heavy flameproof casserole, remove with a slotted spoon, and reserve.

Stir the onion into the casserole and cook gently until soft, adding the garlic toward the end. Stir in the flour and spices for 1 minute, then stir in the stock, citrus zests and juice, spiced vinegar, honey, and

Above: Braised Lamb with Spiced Dried Fruits is a deliciously rich, sweet-sour casserole.

cayenne and season with salt and pepper. Bring to a boil, stirring.

Return the lamb to the casserole, cover tightly, and cook for 1 hour 10 minutes. Stir in the spiced dried fruits, cover, and cook for another 10 minutes or until tender.

Dates, Figs and Mangoes

Low-Sugar Date and Apricot Jam

The concentrated natural sugar in the dried fruits means that little additional sugar is needed in this jam. It is not sufficiently low in overall sugar, however, to be suitable for diabetics.

MAKES ABOUT 3⅓ CUPS

1 pound dried apricot halves
1½ pounds dried dates, pitted and chopped
1¼ cups warmed sugar (see page 7)
juice of 1 lemon
½ cup hazelnuts, chopped

Put the apricots in a nonmetallic bowl, add 2½ cups water, cover, and leave to stand for 12 hours or overnight, until the apricots are plump.

Transfer the contents of the bowl to a large saucepan, add another 2½ cups water and the dates, and simmer until the apricots are soft and tender.

Over low heat, add the warmed sugar and the lemon juice and stir until the sugar has dissolved. Raise the heat and bring to a boil, then reduce the heat and simmer, stirring occasionally, until the jam thickens. Add the hazelnuts and simmer for another 2 minutes.

Remove the pan from the heat and skim off any scum that has formed on the surface with a slotted spoon. Leave the jam to cool for 10–15 minutes, then stir and ladle the jam into warm, clean, dry jars. Cover, seal, and process (see pages 12–13). Leave to cool, then store in a cool, dark, dry place for a few days before eating.

Variations: Use walnuts or almonds instead of hazelnuts; use the juice of an orange instead of a lemon.

Dried Fig and Apple Jam

The fruit in this recipe is easily chopped by hand (I chop both fruits together). If you prefer to remove the fig seeds, press the cooked fruit through a nonmetallic sieve (if you do this, there is no need to peel and core the apples).

MAKES ABOUT 5⅓ CUPS

3 pounds apples, peeled, cored, and finely chopped
1 pound dried figs, stems removed, finely chopped
finely grated zest and juice of 1 large orange
¼ teaspoon ground cinnamon
¼ teaspoon freshly grated nutmeg
pinch of ground cloves
5¾ cups warmed sugar (see page 7)

Put all the ingredients except the sugar in a large saucepan and just cover with water. Bring to a boil, then simmer for 20–30 minutes or until the fruit is completely tender and the liquid well reduced.

Over low heat, add the warmed sugar to the pan and stir the mixture until the sugar has dissolved, then raise the heat and boil for 10–15 minutes, stirring as necessary, until setting point is reached (see page 17).

Remove the pan from the heat and skim the scum from the surface using a slotted spoon. Ladle the jam into warm, clean, dry jars. Cover, seal, and process the jars (see pages 12–13). Leave the jars to cool, then store the jam in a cool, dark, dry place for a few days before eating.

Variation: Use ground allspice or Chinese five-spice powder instead of cinnamon.

Raisin, Date, and Orange Chutney

MAKES ABOUT 4 CUPS

1 pound oranges
1½ pounds dried dates, pitted and chopped
1⅓ cups plump raisins
3 cups chopped onions
3¼ cups sugar
1½ quarts Spiced Vinegar (see page 139)

Finely grate the orange zest and put half into a large saucepan. Remove and discard the orange pith. Chop the oranges, discarding the seeds. Add the oranges and remaining ingredients (except the zest) to the pan.

Bring the mixture to a boil, then simmer for about 1 hour, stirring occasionally, until the chutney has thickened and no free liquid can be seen in the pan.

Stir in the remaining orange zest and ladle the chutney into warm, clean, dry jars; do not trap any air bubbles. Cover with acid-proof lids, seal, and process (see pages 12–13). Store in a cool, dark, dry place for at least 2 months before eating.

Dried Mango Chutney

Cooked dried mangoes have a more pronounced mango flavor than cooked fresh ones, making a fruitier chutney.

MAKES ABOUT 4 CUPS

8 ounces dried mangoes
1 dried red chili, halved
6 cardamom pods, crushed
3 whole cloves
5 allspice berries
1 teaspoon coriander seeds, crushed
1 cinnamon stick, broken in half
12 ounces cooking apples, peeled, cored, and chopped
1 garlic clove, cut into slivers

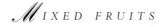

sea salt
1¼ cups white wine vinegar
1¾ cups warmed sugar (see page 7)

Place the mangoes in a nonmetallic bowl, just cover them with water, and leave to soak overnight. Drain off the soaking liquid and boil the liquid until reduced to 1¼ cups.

Gently heat the chili and spices in a dry heavy skillet until fragrant, moving them around gently so that they do not burn, then add to the pan along with the apples, mangoes, garlic, a good pinch of salt, and the vinegar. Bring to a boil, then simmer for about 10 minutes, stirring occasionally.

Over low heat, stir in the warmed sugar until it has dissolved. Raise the heat and boil, stirring frequently, until the chutney is thick and no free liquid is visible.

Spoon into warm, clean, dry jars, taking care not to trap any air bubbles. Cover with acid-proof lids, seal, and process (see pages 12–13). Store in a cool, dark, dry place for 1 month before eating.

Mostarda di Frutta

This is a tongue-tingling combination!

MAKES ABOUT 1⅔ CUPS

1 cup dry English mustard
10 tablespoons light brown sugar
¾ cup white wine vinegar
⅔ cup each dried apricot halves, dried figs,
**   raisins, and glacé cherries, coarsely chopped**
⅓ cup dried apple rings, quartered
6 pieces of preserved ginger in syrup
1 teaspoon sea salt

In a bowl, stir 1¼ cups water into the mustard. Cover and leave for at least 1 hour.

Place the sugar and vinegar in a saucepan and heat gently, stirring, until the sugar has dissolved. Raise the heat to moderate and boil until the mixture begins to thicken.

Stir in the fruits, ginger, salt, and dissolved mustard and return to a boil, stirring. Simmer until the mixture is quite thick. Leave to cool, then spoon into clean, dry jars; it is important that you do not trap any air bubbles. Cover with acid-proof lids, seal, and process (see pages 12–13). Store in a cool, dark, dry place for 6–8 weeks before eating.

Serving Suggestion
In Lombardy, Mostarda di Frutta is the classic accompaniment to boiled meats, but I suggest you serve it with broiled and roast poultry and meats.

Below: Mostarda di Frutta is an unusual traditional preserve from Lombardy in Italy.

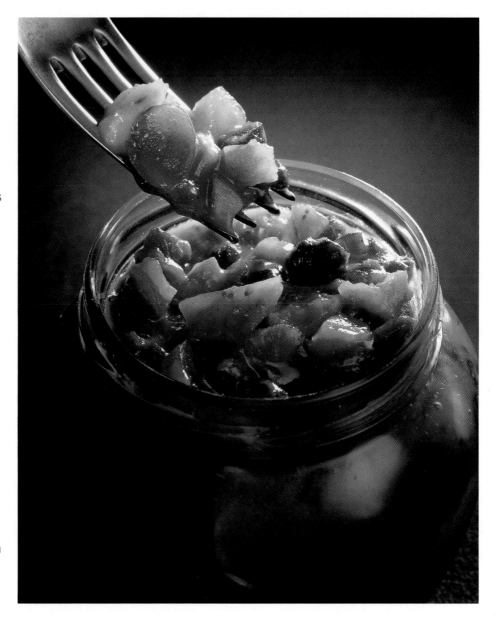

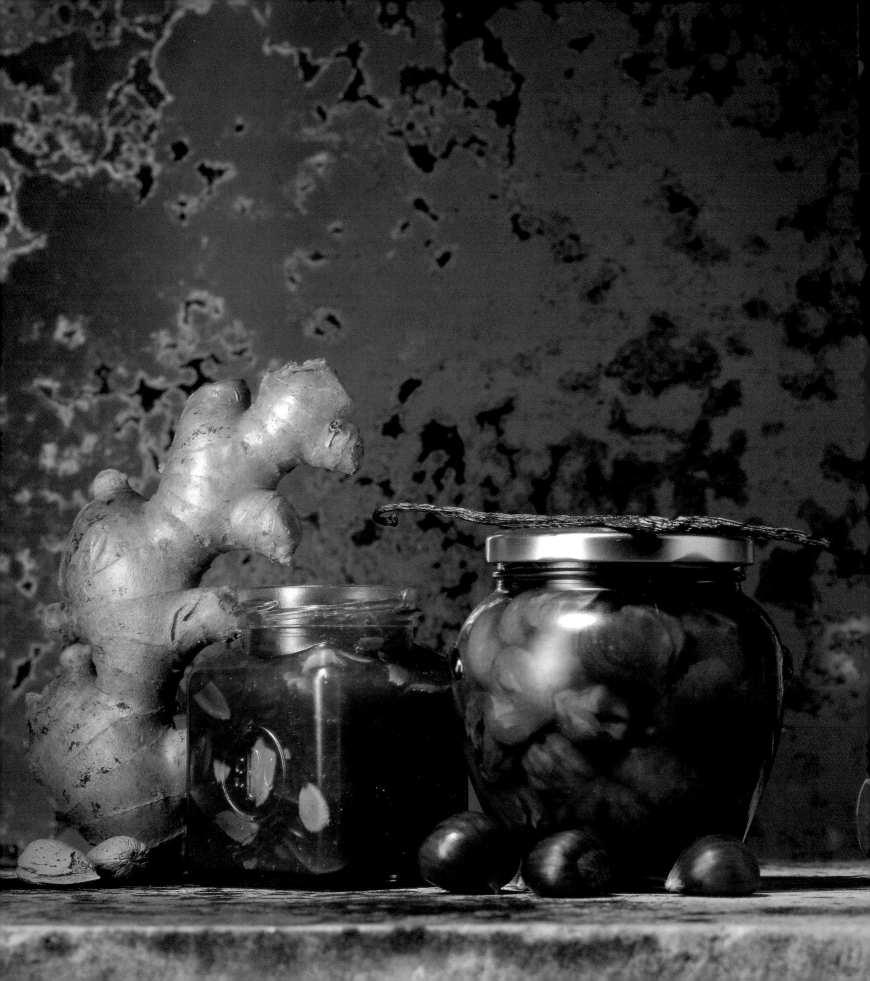

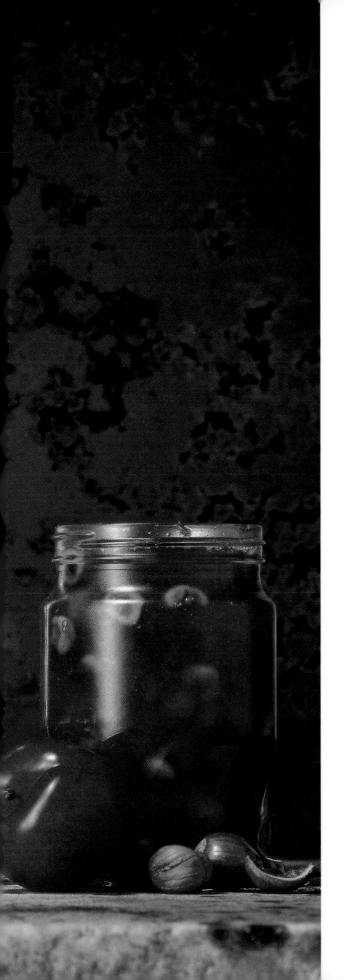

$\mathscr{N}$ U T S

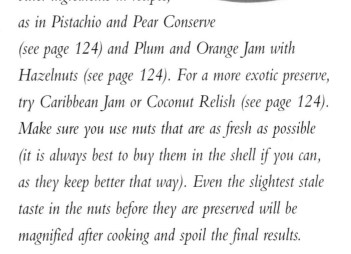

As well as adding flavor to numerous sweet and savory preserves, nuts also provide an interesting texture. Nuts can be the main attraction of a preserve, such as the chestnuts in Chestnut, Vanilla, and Rum Jam (see page 122), or they may play a complementary role with other ingredients in recipes, as in Pistachio and Pear Conserve (see page 124) and Plum and Orange Jam with Hazelnuts (see page 124). For a more exotic preserve, try Caribbean Jam or Coconut Relish (see page 124). Make sure you use nuts that are as fresh as possible (it is always best to buy them in the shell if you can, as they keep better that way). Even the slightest stale taste in the nuts before they are preserved will be magnified after cooking and spoil the final results.

Left (from left to right): Almond, Carrot, and Ginger Chutney, Chestnuts in Syrup, and Plum and Orange Jam with Hazelnuts.

Almond, Carrot, and Ginger Chutney

The carrots can be grated lengthwise, crosswise, or diagonally, depending on how long you like the strands to be.

MAKES ABOUT 3⅓ CUPS

4 cups grated carrots
2 tablespoons plus 1 teaspoon ground coriander
2 tablespoons sea salt
generous pinch of cayenne pepper
finely grated zest and juice of 1 lemon
1 cup cider vinegar
2 ounces fresh ginger, peeled
1¾ cups warmed sugar (see page 7)
3 tablespoons clear honey
generous ⅓ cup sliced almonds

Put the carrots, coriander, salt, cayenne pepper, lemon zest and juice, and vinegar into a nonmetallic bowl. Grate half the ginger and cut the other half into matchsticks. Stir all the ginger into the bowl, then cover and leave in a cool place overnight.

Transfer the contents of the bowl to a large saucepan. Add ⅔ cup water and bring to a boil, then simmer for 20 minutes. Over low heat, stir in the warmed sugar and honey until both have dissolved, then return to a boil. Simmer for another 20–25 minutes, stirring as necessary, until the mixture is thick and no free liquid is visible. Stir in the almonds and simmer the mixture for another 4 minutes or so.

Remove from the heat and ladle into warm, clean, dry jars, taking care not to trap any air bubbles. Cover with acid-proof lids, seal, and process (see pages 12–13). Allow to mature for at least a few days, preferably much longer, before eating.

Chestnuts in Syrup

Peeling chestnuts is a laborious task, but don't be tempted to use reconstituted dried chestnuts – you will be very disappointed with the end result. You need to end up with 12 ounces prepared nuts. Glucose can be bought from a pharmacy.

MAKES ABOUT 1 CUP

1½ pounds chestnuts
1 vanilla bean
1¼ cups sugar
¾ cup liquid glucose
2 tablespoons brandy or dark rum (optional)

Make a slit in the shell of each chestnut, then add them to a pan of boiling water and simmer for 10 minutes. Remove the pan from the heat and, using a slotted spoon, remove the nuts, one by one. When they are cool enough to handle, remove both the shell and the fine inner skin (see below).

Simmer the chestnuts and vanilla bean in just enough water to cover for about 5 minutes or until tender but not breaking up. Drain and dry on paper towels; reserve the vanilla bean.

Gently heat the sugar, glucose, and ¾ cup water in a pan large enough to hold the

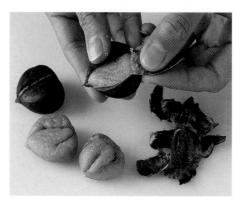

Peeling chestnuts: When preparing chestnuts, be sure to remove the fine inner skin as well as the tough outer shell.

chestnuts, stirring until the sugar and glucose have dissolved. Raise the heat and bring to a boil. Remove from the heat and add the chestnuts, then return to a boil. Take off the heat again, then cover and leave overnight.

The next day, uncover the pan and boil the chestnuts in the syrup once more. Remove the pan from the heat, cover, and once more leave overnight. The following day, add the vanilla bean and boil for the last time. Off the heat, stir in the brandy or dark rum if using, then pour the chestnuts and syrup into a warm, clean, dry jar. Rotate the jar to expel any air bubbles. Cover, seal, and process (see pages 12–13). Store in a cool, dark, dry place.

Serving Suggestion
Serve for dessert with crème fraîche, ice cream, or thick yogurt; serve with chocolate soufflés, chocolate cake, or other chocolate desserts; serve with crème caramel.

Chestnut, Vanilla, and Rum Jam

This is a superior version of the *crème de marrons* that is sold in small jars. I like to use light brown sugar for this recipe.

MAKES ABOUT 4 CUPS

about 2¾ pounds chestnuts
1 vanilla bean
3 cups soft brown sugar, warmed (see page 7)
2 tablespoons dark rum

Prepare the chestnuts as for Chestnuts in Syrup (see left).

Put the nuts and vanilla bean in a large saucepan and add just enough water to cover. Cover the pan and bring to a boil, then simmer for about 30 minutes or until

$\mathscr{C}$HESTNUTS

the chestnuts are tender. Drain the chestnuts, reserving the liquid. Remove the vanilla bean from the chestnuts, then purée the nuts in a blender or food processor. Measure the purée; there should be about 2⅔ cups in total.

Split the vanilla bean lengthwise and scrape out the seeds. Put the bean and seeds in a heavy pan and add the chestnut purée, sugar, and 7 tablespoons reserved cooking liquid. Heat gently, stirring, until the sugar has dissolved, then boil until the mixture is thick. Discard the vanilla bean and stir in the rum.

Spoon the jam into warm, clean, dry jars, cover, seal, and process (see pages 12–13). Leave overnight to cool and set slightly. This delicious jam will keep for about 6 months in a cool, dark, dry place.

Serving Suggestion
Use to sandwich chocolate cakes together or to fill a chocolate Swiss roll; spoon into meringue baskets, top with a swirl of whipped cream, and decorate with plenty of dark chocolate shavings; fill chocolate crêpes; stir into crème anglaise, crème pâtissière, or whipped cream; use as the base for soufflés, mousses, and ice creams; mix with whipped cream, crème fraîche, or yogurt to make a quick chestnut fool (see right); serve with lightly sweetened poached orange slices or kumquats.

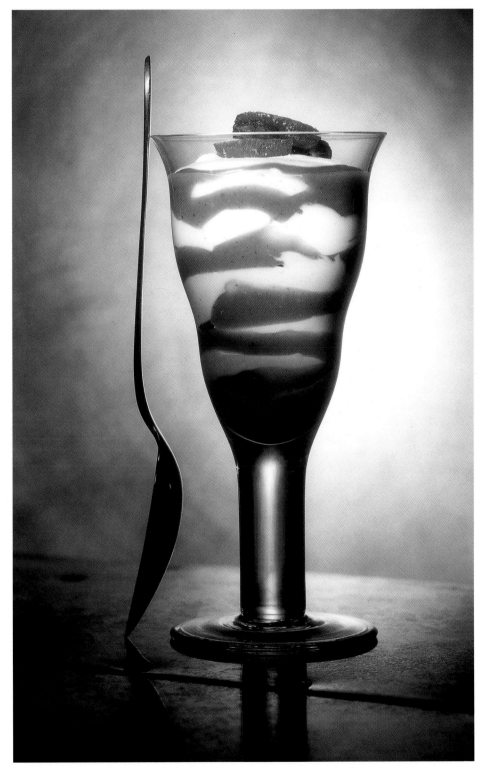

Right: Use Chestnut, Vanilla, and Rum Jam layered with cream, crème fraîche, or thick yogurt to make a delicious chestnut fool.

Caribbean Jam

An exotic jam to make for special occasions or special people.

MAKES ABOUT 4 CUPS

1 coconut
6 limes
1 pineapple
2 cooking apples, chopped but not peeled or cored
4½ cups warmed sugar (see page 7)

Pierce the eyes of the coconut with a sharp metal skewer and drain the liquid into a large saucepan. Crack open the coconut with a hammer and cut the flesh away from the shell. Coarsely grate the flesh and add it to the pan. Grate the lime zest and set aside. Squeeze the juice from the limes (reserve the lime halves) and add to the pan. Chop the lime halves and put these in the pan.

Peel the pineapple, making sure you remove all the eyes and reserving the peel. Chop the flesh quite finely and mix with the lime zest. Chop the pineapple peel and put into the pan with the apples and 1¼ quarts water. Bring to a boil, cover, and simmer steadily for about 1 hour.

Strain the boiled juice into a clean pan, pressing down well on the lime peels. Add the pineapple flesh and lime zest to the pan and simmer for about 20 minutes, stirring occasionally, until the pineapple is tender.

Over low heat, stir in the warmed sugar until it has dissolved. Raise the heat and boil vigorously for 10–15 minutes, stirring as necessary, until setting point is reached (see page 17).

Remove from the heat and skim the surface with a slotted spoon. Ladle into warm, clean, dry jars. Cover, seal, and process (see pages 12–13). Leave overnight to set. Store in a cool, dark, dry place.

Serving Suggestion
Delicious with toast or added to plain yogurt.

Coconut Relish

This recipe was given to me by the daughter-in-law of a neighbor. When I told this neighbor I was writing a book on preserving, she told me her daughter-in-law had an "interesting" relish recipe that she would get for me. Unlike many things that are described as interesting because nothing else that isn't derogatory can be said about them, this crunchy pickle is indeed very good.

MAKES ABOUT 2 CUPS

1 coconut
½ teaspoon ground ginger
1 cinnamon stick
good pinch of cayenne powder
1 large onion (not Spanish), finely chopped
2–3 garlic cloves, chopped
5–10 tablespoons sugar
1 teaspoon sea salt
1¼ cups cider vinegar

Pierce the eyes of the coconut with a sharp metal skewer and pour the liquid into a pan. Crack open the coconut with a hammer and cut the flesh away from the shell. Coarsely grate the flesh and add it to the pan with the remaining ingredients.

Bring to a boil, stirring, cover the pan, and simmer for 30 minutes. Remove the lid and boil for about 15 minutes, stirring occasionally, until the liquid has reduced and the relish has thickened.

Remove the chutney from the heat and ladle into warm, clean, dry jars. Cover with acid-proof lids, seal, and process (see pages 12–13). Store in a cool, dark, dry place for at least 1 month before using.

Serving Suggestion
Serve with curries and other spicy meat, poultry, and fish dishes.

Pistachio and Pear Conserve

The delicate flavor of pistachios goes well with the gentle flavor of pears, and the nuts add pretty flecks of green.

MAKES ABOUT 4 CUPS

2¼ pounds pears, peeled, cored, and cubed
juice of 1 lemon
5¾ cups warmed sugar (see page 7)
¾ cup coarsely chopped pistachios

Put the pears, lemon juice, and 1¼ cups water into a large saucepan and bring to a boil. Lower the heat and simmer for 10 minutes or until the pears are tender.

Add the sugar to the pan and stir over low heat until the sugar has dissolved. Raise the heat and boil vigorously for 15–20 minutes, stirring occasionally, until the mixture has thickened slightly.

Remove the pan from the heat and skim any scum from the surface, then stir in the nuts. Leave to stand for 10–15 minutes, then stir and ladle into warm, clean, dry jars, taking care not to trap any air bubbles. Cover, seal, and process (see pages 12–13). Leave overnight to set slightly. Store in a cool, dark, dry place.

Plum and Orange Jam with Hazelnuts

Lightly toasted chopped hazelnuts add both flavor and texture to this popular jam.

MAKES ABOUT 4 CUPS

2¼ pounds plums, pitted
finely grated zest and juice of 1 small orange or 1 lime
1 cup hazelnuts
5 cups sugar

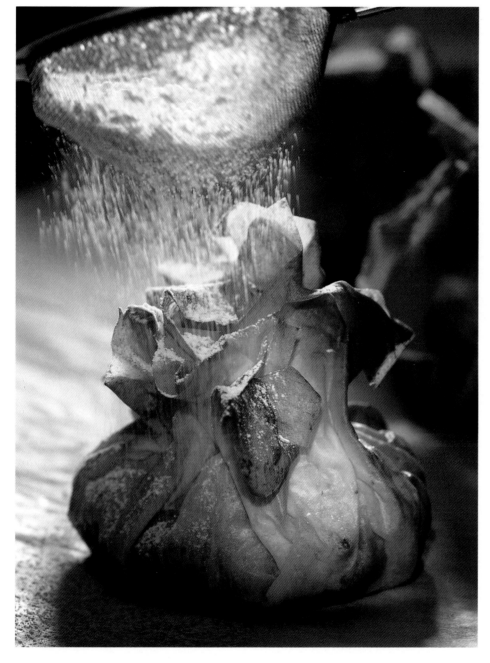

Left: Brush sheets of phyllo pastry with melted butter. Top with spoonfuls of Pecan and Whiskey Mincemeat, then twist the corners of each sheet together. Bake for 10 minutes at 400°F. Dust with confectioners' sugar, and serve.

the heat and boil vigorously for 10–15 minutes, stirring as necessary, until setting point is reached (see page 17).

Remove from the heat. Skim the scum from the surface with a slotted spoon. Leave to stand for 10–15 minutes, then stir and ladle into warm, clean, dry jars. Cover, seal, and process (see pages 12–13). Leave overnight to set. Store in a cool, dark, dry place.

Pecan and Whiskey Mincemeat

MAKES ABOUT 3⅓ CUPS

1 cup chopped pecans
12 ounces cooking apples, peeled, cored, and finely chopped
1⅓ cups plump raisins
⅔ cup finely chopped dried apricot halves
scant ⅔ cup each finely chopped pitted dates and dried figs
1 cup golden raisins
1 teaspoon freshly grated nutmeg
1 teaspoon ground cinnamon
pinch of ground allspice
¾ cup shredded beef or vegetable suet
10 tablespoons dark brown sugar
finely grated zest and juice of 2 oranges
finely grated zest and juice of 1 lemon
1¼ cups whiskey

Stir together all the ingredients in a nonmetallic bowl. Cover and leave in a cool place for 24 hours, stirring occasionally.

Pack tightly into clean, dry jars, pressing down to expel any air. Cover, seal, and process (see pages 12–13). Store in a cool, dark, dry place for 6–8 weeks before using.

Put the plums in a large saucepan with ⅓ cup water and the orange or lime juice and zest. Bring to a boil, then simmer for about 20 minutes or until the fruit is soft. Meanwhile, preheat the broiler. Spread the hazelnuts in a single layer on a baking sheet and toast until the skins split and the nuts begin to brown; stir as necessary so that they brown evenly. Transfer to a colander and rub with a cloth to remove the skins. Chop the nuts. Stir the sugar and nuts into the plums until the sugar has dissolved. Raise

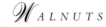

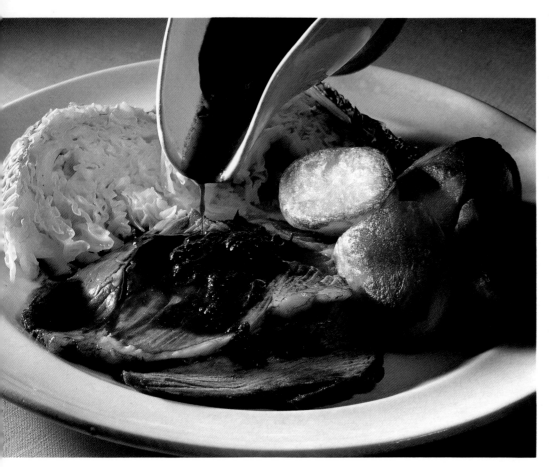

Roast Beef with Pickled Walnut Sauce

The slightly piquant, rich flavor of this sauce is a fitting companion for good roast beef.

SERVES 6

1 piece of rib roast on the bone, about 5 pounds
mild olive oil for brushing
freshly ground black pepper
6 Pickled Walnuts (see left), drained
1½ cups red wine
about ⅓ cup stock, preferably beef
1 tablespoon unsalted butter
salt

Preheat the oven to 450°F.

Weigh the roast to calculate the cooking time, then brush with oil and sprinkle with black pepper – do not add salt. Put the roast on a rack in a roasting pan. Roast for 10–12 minutes, then lower the oven temperature to 350°F and roast for 12–15 minutes per 1 pound for rare, 15–18 minutes for medium-rare, or 18–20 minutes for well-done. Baste the meat occasionally with the pan juices. Turn off the oven. Remove the roast from the oven and let stand for 10 minutes at room temperature while you make the sauce.

Pour off almost all the fat from the roasting pan, leaving behind the pan juices. Add the pickled walnuts to the pan juices, mashing them with a fork, then stir in the wine. Bring to a boil, stir in the stock, and boil until concentrated.

Over low heat, gradually stir in the butter, making sure each piece is incorporated before the next is added. Season with salt and pepper and pour into a warm sauceboat to serve with the beef.

Pickled Walnuts

MAKES ABOUT 2 QUARTS

1 pound green walnuts
10 tablespoons table salt
1½ ounces fresh ginger
7½ cups white wine vinegar
¾ cup black peppercorns
6 tablespoons allspice berries

Prick the nuts well all over with an embroidery needle and put them in a nonmetallic bowl. Dissolve half the salt in 2½ cups water, pour over the nuts, cover, and leave in a cool place for 1 week.

Drain off and throw away the soaking liquid. Next, dissolve the remaining salt in 2½ cups water. Pour this over the nuts,

Above: Roast Beef with Pickled Walnut Sauce make a fine pair for a special dinner.

and leave the bowl in a cool place for another 2 weeks.

Drain the walnuts (discarding the liquid), rinse, and dry. Spread out the nuts and leave exposed to the air for 2–3 weeks or until they have turned black. Pack them into clean, dry jars.

Bruise the ginger with the flat side of a knife, place in a large pan with the vinegar, peppercorns and allspice, and boil for 10 minutes. Pour the liquid over the nuts. Rotate to expel air bubbles. Leave to cool. Cover with acid-proof lids, seal, and process (see pages 12–13). Store in a cool, dark, dry place for 1 month before using.

𝒲ALNUTS AND 𝒜LMONDS

Walnut, Apple, and Date Chutney

Walnuts give this chutney a crunchy texture and a delicious nutty flavor that complements the fruity taste of apples and dried dates.

MAKES 5⅓ CUPS

1 pound onions, chopped
2 pounds crisp, tart cooking apples, peeled, cored and chopped
¾ cup walnuts, chopped
1½ pounds dried dates, pitted and chopped
1 teaspoon ground ginger
1 teaspoon cayenne pepper
1 teaspoon salt
1½ cups white wine vinegar
2 cups light brown sugar

Put the onions in a heavy saucepan and add a little water. Bring to a boil, then cover and simmer until the onions are tender.

Add the apples and cook, covered, over low heat for another 15–20 minutes, shaking the pan occasionally, until the apples are almost tender.

Stir in the walnuts, dates, ginger, cayenne pepper, salt, and half of the vinegar. Boil gently, uncovered, stirring occasionally, until the chutney thickens.

Over low heat, add the sugar and remaining vinegar and stir until the sugar has dissolved. Raise the heat and boil, stirring as necessary, until the chutney is thick and there is no free liquid.

Ladle into warm, clean, dry jars. Cover with acid-proof lids, seal, and process (see pages 12–13). Store in a cool, dark, dry place for 1 month before eating.

Serving Suggestion
Serve with pork, ham, cold meat pies, and cheeses (the chutney gives a real fillip to cheese sandwiches).

Almond Plum Sauce

If you use yellow plums and white sugar to make this recipe your sauce will be golden in colour, whereas dark plums and brown sugar will produce a denser, purplish-red sauce.

MAKES ABOUT 3¾ CUPS

2 pounds plums, chopped
2 cups white or light brown sugar
1 teaspoon ground ginger
8 whole cloves
a few drops of Tabasco sauce
1 teaspoon sea salt
2½ cups white or red wine vinegar
⅓ cup silvered almonds

Put all the ingredients except the almonds into a large saucepan. Heat gently, stirring, until the sugar has dissolved. Bring to a boil, then simmer gently, uncovered, for about 30 minutes, stirring occasionally, until the plums have softened.

Pour the contents of the saucepan into a nonmetallic sieve placed over a clean

Left: The green walnuts used for Pickled Walnuts should be picked before the hard shells form; this is usually at the end of June.

saucepan. Using a wooden spoon, press the contents of the sieve to make sure as much sauce as possible is squeezed through.

Simmer the sauce, uncovered, stirring as necessary, until it has the consistency of heavy cream. Pour into warm, clean, dry bottles, cover with acid-proof lids, seal, and process (see pages 12–13). Store in a cool, dark, dry place for 1 month before serving.

Serving Suggestion
Serve with hot or cold game and cold game pies, chicken, turkey and duck, cold cuts, and sharp cheeses such as Cheddar.

Almond, Plum, and Rum Jam

Almonds have a natural affinity with plums; their subtle flavor highlights the richness of the fruit.

MAKES ABOUT 5⅓ CUPS

2 pounds plums, pitted
½ cup plump raisins
1¼ cups water
1½ pounds warmed sugar
2 tablespoons dark rum
½ cup almonds, chopped

Put the plums, raisins and water in a large saucepan and simmer gently, uncovered, shaking the pan frequently, for about 20 minutes or until the plums are soft.

Over low heat, add the sugar and stir until it has dissolved. Raise the heat and boil for about 15 minutes, stirring as necessary, until setting point is reached (see page 17).

Remove the pan from the heat and stir in the rum. Let stand about 15 minutes, then stir in the almonds. Ladle the mixture into warm, clean, dry jars. Cover, seal, and process (see pages 12–13). Leave overnight to set. Store in a cool, dark, dry place.

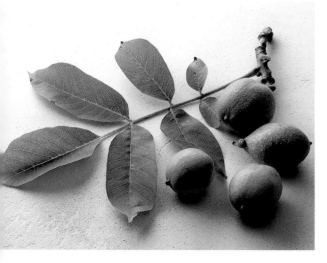

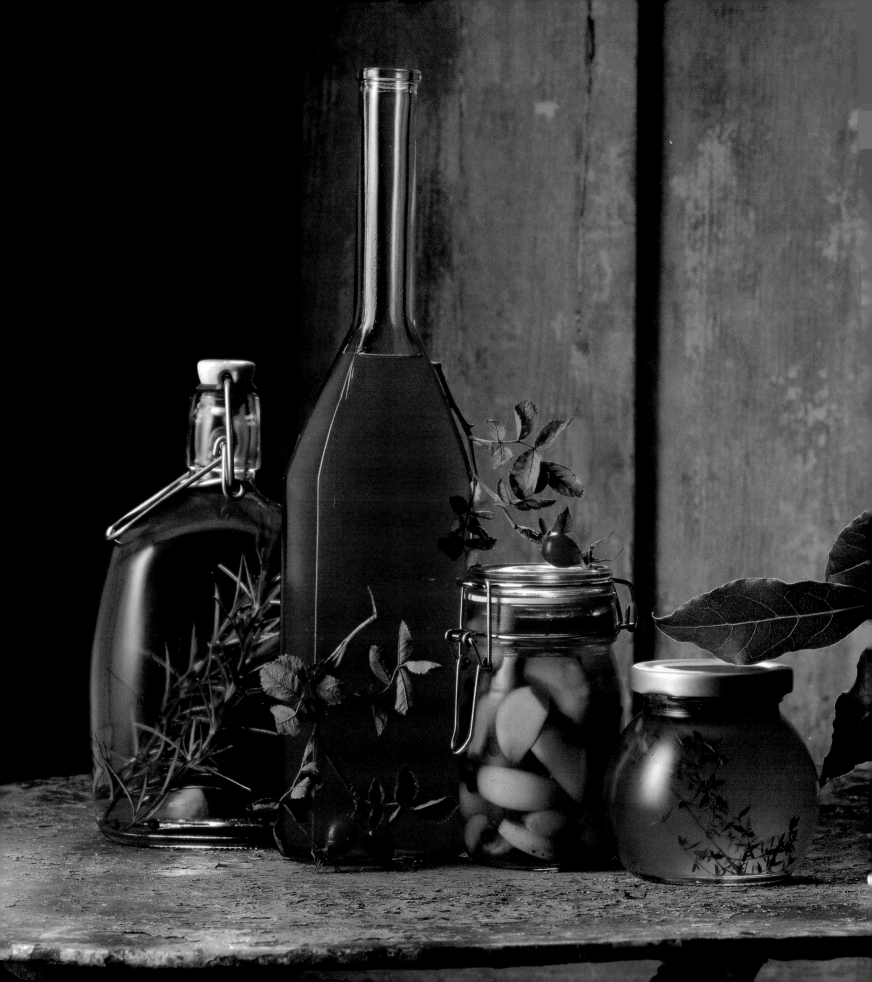

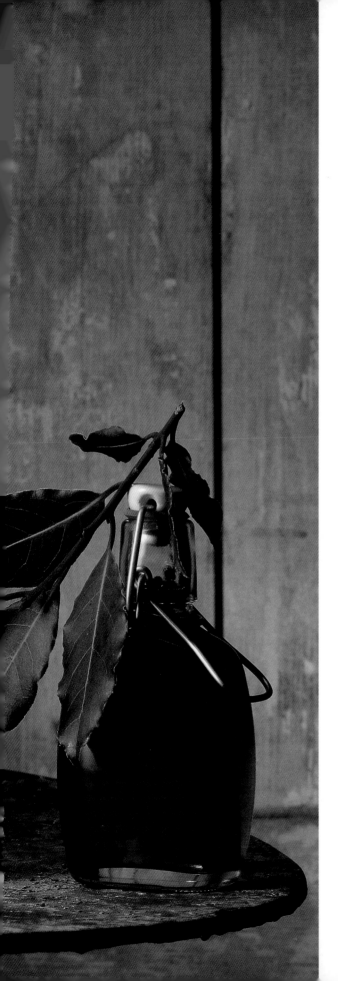

FLOWERS, HERBS, AND AROMATICS

The subtle yet pervasive scents of flowers, herbs, and aromatics give an enticingly unusual taste and aroma to a variety of different preserves. Flowers, herbs, and aromatics can be used as the main ingredient of a preserve, such as Elderflower Cordial (see page 130), or they 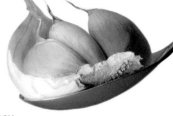 can lend a vital supporting role to other ingredients, giving them new life, as in recipes like Rhubarb and Ginger Conserve (see page 135) and Old-fashioned Rose Petal Vinegar (see page 138). Avoid using any flowers and herbs that have been treated with chemicals or those growing by the roadside. For flowers and herbs in peak condition, pick them in the morning of a dry day, after the dew has evaporated but before the sun is hot. Always pick herbs before they have flowered.

Left (from left to right): Herb Oil, Rose Hip Syrup, Saffron Garlic, Herb Jelly, and Spiced Vinegar.

129

CARNATIONS, ELDERFLOWERS AND ELDERBERRIES

Carnation Liqueur

Of the various carnations, the only one to use for this liqueur is *Dianthus caryophyllus*, the clove pink of English country gardens.

MAKES ABOUT 1 QUART

5 ounces carnation heads
1 whole clove
1-inch piece cinnamon stick
2½ cups vodka
1¼ cups sugar

Lightly bruise the carnations with the end of a rolling pin, then pack them into a wide-necked bottle with the spices.

Gently warm the vodka in a large saucepan, then pour into the bottle. Cover and leave in a warm place for 2 months, shaking the bottle every other day.

Pour the contents of the bottle into a sieve lined with a double thickness of cheesecloth and leave to drain for a few hours.

Gently heat the sugar in 1¼ cups water, stirring, until the sugar has dissolved, then leave to cool.

Mix the flavored vodka with the sugar syrup, then pour into a clean, dry bottle. Cover and seal (see pages 12–13). This is now ready to drink.

Elderflower Cordial

Making this cordial is a sign that summer should be here very soon. This is really the best way of preserving elderflowers, as they turn brown and limp when frozen.

MAKES ABOUT 1¼ QUARTS

about 15 large elderflower umbels (heads)
4½ cups sugar
1 lemon, sliced
1½ ounces citric acid
2¼ cups water, boiling

Put the elderflowers, sugar, lemon slices, and citric acid in a large heatproof bowl and stir in the water to dissolve the sugar. Cover and leave in a cool place for 4 days, stirring occasionally; taste to see if the flavor is strong enough, remembering that the cordial will be diluted for drinking.

Strain through a nonmetallic sieve lined with cheesecloth and pour into bottles. Seal and process (see pages 12–13) and keep in a cool, dark, dry place. This cordial is ready to drink and will keep for a very long time.

Serving Suggestion
Drink chilled, diluted with water or dry white wine; add to fruit desserts such as gooseberry, strawberry, peach, or raspberry tarts; use to flavor creamy desserts.

Gooseberry and Elderflower Butter

Gooseberries and luscious muscat-flavored elderflowers make an ideal partnership. Both are seasonal, but fortuitously, nature has devised that the two seasons coincide. Made lightly fragrant by the flowers, this soft, thick, "buttery" spread is the perfect vehicle for this heavenly combination.

MAKES ABOUT 3⅓ CUPS

3 pounds gooseberries
3 elderflower umbels (heads)
warmed sugar (see page 7)

Put the gooseberries, elderflowers, and ⅔ cup water in a large saucepan and simmer gently until the fruit is very soft and pulpy.

Push through a nonmetallic sieve with a wooden spoon. Measure the purée and return to the rinsed pan with 1¾ cups sugar for every 2½ cups purée.

Heat gently, stirring, until the sugar has dissolved, then increase the heat and boil slowly for 30–45 minutes, stirring frequently, until the mixture is as thick as sour cream.

Spoon into warm, clean, dry jars. Cover, seal, and process (see pages 12–13). Store the butter in a cool, dark, dry place for a few days before eating.

Serving Suggestion
Use to fill layer cakes; fill small, crisp tartlet shells and top with lightly poached gooseberries; or spread on scones or not-too-thin slices of freshly cut good-quality white bread.

Elderberry Sauce

Make the most of dark, fragrant elderberries while they are in season by making this delicious, subtly spicy sauce.

MAKES ABOUT 5 CUPS

3 whole cloves
2 allspice berries
5 black peppercorns
¼-inch piece cinnamon stick
1 dried red chili
1¼ cups red wine vinegar
2 pounds elderberries
1 onion, chopped
2 cups sugar
2 teaspoons sea salt

Place the cloves, allspice berries, peppercorns, cinnamon stick, and chili on a square of cheesecloth and tie with string to make a small bag. Add the cheesecloth bag to a large saucepan with the vinegar, cover the pan, and bring the vinegar to a boil. Remove from the heat and leave overnight, covered, in a cool place.

Add the elderberries, onion, sugar, and salt to the vinegar and simmer for 10–15 minutes or until the elderberries are tender. Remove the cheesecloth bag from the pan and strain the sauce through a nonmetallic

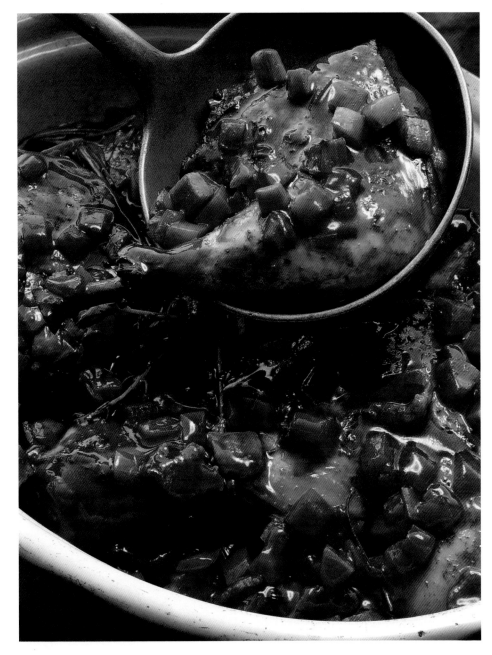

Pheasant and Elderberry Casserole

The first time I made this recipe I prepared it by the method given below. The second time I put everything in a heavy nonmetallic casserole, left it to marinate overnight, then put it straight in the oven. Although the first result was better, the second casserole was quite acceptable. The cooking time in the oven will depend on the age of the bird.

SERVES 2

1 pheasant, cut into 4 pieces
small handful of fresh herbs, such as parsley, thyme, rosemary, and chives
salt and freshly ground black pepper
1½ cups medium-bodied red wine
1 tablespoon oil
4 ounces thick-cut bacon, chopped
1 onion, chopped
2 carrots, chopped
2 tablespoons Elderberry Sauce (see page 130)

Put the pheasant, herbs, and seasonings in a nonmetallic bowl, add the wine, cover, and place in the refrigerator for about 8 hours, turning the bird over occasionally.

Preheat the oven to 300°F. Remove the pheasant from the wine and dry thoroughly. Reserve the wine.

Heat the oil in a heavy flameproof casserole, add the bacon, and cook until it is beginning to brown and the fat has been rendered. Add the onion and carrots and cook until lightly browned. Remove with a slotted spoon. Add the pieces of pheasant and brown lightly. Remove. Stir the wine with the herbs into the casserole and bring to a boil. Add the elderberry sauce. Return the pheasant, vegetables, and bacon to the casserole. Cover and bake until the pheasant is tender. If the sauce is not concentrated enough, remove the pheasant and keep warm, then boil the sauce until sufficiently reduced.

sieve into a bowl. Return the sauce to the pan and cook over moderate heat, stirring as necessary, until thickened. Pour into warm, clean, dry bottles and cover with acid-proof lids. Process in a water bath for 30 minutes (see page 13).

Above: This Pheasant and Elderberry Casserole makes use of aromatic Elderberry Sauce, producing a richly flavored dish that is simple to prepare.

Rose Hip Syrup

According to an old English tradition, if rose hips are to be used in cooking, they should be picked after the first frost has hit them.

Rose hip syrup is very rich in vitamin C, which is destroyed by heat, so the syrup is not made by the same method as other syrups but in a way that preserves the vitamin. Once opened, the syrup will not keep for more than a week or two, so it is best to fill only small bottles.

MAKES ABOUT 2½ CUPS

2 pounds ripe rose hips
2¼ cups warmed sugar (see page 7)

Bring 7½ cups water to a boil. Meanwhile, coarsely chop the rose hips, then immediately add to the water. Return to a boil and remove from the heat, then leave to infuse for 15 minutes.

Pour the contents of the pan into a scalded jelly bag suspended over a bowl and leave for 8–12 hours or until most of the juice has strained through.

Return the rose hips in the jelly bag to the saucepan, add 3½ cups water and bring to a boil. Remove from the heat and leave for 10 minutes, then pour the contents of the pan back into the jelly bag and leave to strain again into the bowl for 4–6 hours.

Pour the juice into the rinsed pan and simmer until reduced to about 3½ cups.

Over low heat, stir the warmed sugar into the juice until it has dissolved. Raise the heat and boil for 5 minutes. Pour the syrup into hot bottles, cover, and seal lightly. Process in a boiling water bath for 5 minutes (see page 13). Remove the bottles from the water bath and tighten the lids immediately. The syrup will keep for up to 1 year.

Serving Suggestion
About 2 teaspoons of the syrup a day is a pleasant, natural, and inexpensive way of boosting the vitamin C content of the diet.

This syrup is also good poured over sponge cake, stirred into fruit salads, and poured over poached fruits.

Crystallized Rose Petals

Home-prepared crystallized rose petals look much better than bought ones. Egg white is sometimes used in place of gum arabic, but I find that gum arabic, which is available from pharmacies and cake-decoration specialty shops, is easier to apply to delicate petals and preserves them better and for a longer time. Other edible flower petals or small leaves, such as mint leaves, can be treated in the same way to use for decorating desserts, cakes, and sweets.

6 large, fragrant roses
1 teaspoon gum arabic
about 3 teaspoons rosewater
superfine sugar

Separate the rose petals before carefully removing all of the white heels, or bases. Dissolve the gum arabic in the rosewater.

Using an artist's or a make-up brush, gently brush the gum arabic solution over

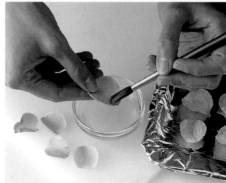

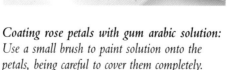

Coating rose petals with gum arabic solution: Use a small brush to paint solution onto the petals, being careful to cover them completely.

3 or 4 petals at a time to cover completely. Dust with an even coating of sugar, making sure there are no patches left bare.

Leave on a foil-lined tray in a warm, dry, airy place, turning carefully, until quite dry. Store on tissue paper or paper towels inside an airtight container. These will stay fresh for at least 1 year.

Rose Petal Jam

In the story of the Arabian Nights, the Caliph of Baghdad had seven palaces, the seventh and most sumptuous being the Palace of Eternal and Unsatiating Delights. At the feasts held there, one of the dishes that was served was a rose petal jam, the honeyed sweetness of which was supposed to have a secret power that held captive anyone who ate it. This jam may or may not be the same as that served at the palace, but it is certainly captivating. It is more like a thick syrup; if you would prefer a firmer set, add commercial liquid pectin or pectin extract (see page 7) with the remaining sugar, then boil for just 4 minutes.

MAKES ABOUT 1⅓ CUPS

8 ounces dark red, very fragrant roses
2¼ cups sugar
juice of 2 lemons
rosewater to taste (optional)

Separate the rose petals, cut off the white heels, or bases, and chop the petals into small but not too fine pieces. Put the chopped petals in a bowl and stir in half the sugar. Cover the bowl and leave for about 24 hours.

In a large saucepan, gently heat the remaining sugar in 5 cups water and the lemon juice, stirring, until the sugar has dissolved. Add the rose petal mixture, raise the heat slightly, and simmer gently for 20 minutes, stirring occasionally.

$\mathcal{R}$OSES

Boil the petal mixture for 5 minutes or until it is thickened but has not reached setting point. Add rosewater if the flavor is not strong enough. Ladle into warm, clean, dry jars. Cover, seal, and process (see pages 12–13). Leave overnight to cool and set. Store in a cool, dark, dry place.

Rose Petal Sorbet

Even in winter, it's easy to conjure up images of an old-fashioned country cottage garden on a summer's afternoon with this delicate sorbet, decorated with crystallized rose petals.

SERVES 4

1¼ cups sugar
about 3 tablespoons Rose Petal Jam
  (see page 132)
liquid red food coloring (optional)
Crystallized Rose Petals (see page 132)
  for decoration

Put the sugar and 3½ cups water in a saucepan and heat gently, stirring, until all the sugar has dissolved. Stir in the rose petal jam, raise the heat, and boil until the mixture is syrupy (similar to the thickness of the syrup in canned fruits). Taste for rose flavor, remembering that freezing will mute it, and add more jam if necessary.

Pour the mixture into a shallow freezer container and leave to cool. Cover and chill in the refrigerator. Transfer to the freezer until just beginning to freeze. Remove from the freezer and pour into a chilled bowl. Whisk with a cold whisk to break up the ice crystals. Whisk in a little food coloring if the color seems too pale. Return to the freezer and repeat once more, sealing the container tightly before final freezing. Serve decorated with a few of the crystallized rose petals.

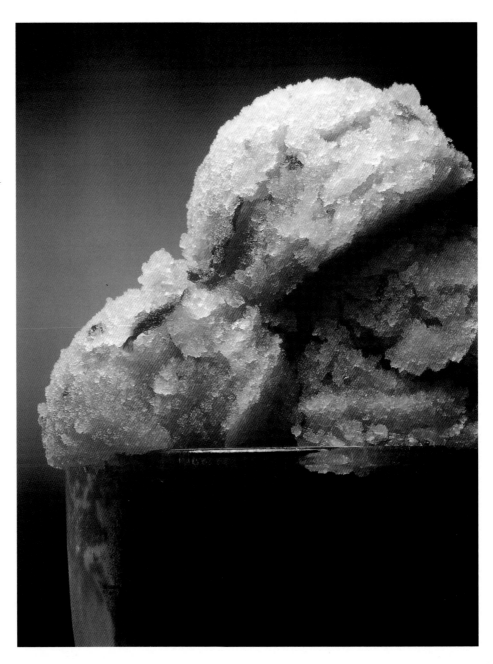

Serving Suggestion
This unusual sorbet is delightful served on its own or accompanied by *langues de chat* or delicate, crisp cookies. Serve in attractive glass bowls.

Above: This fragrant, subtly pink Rose Petal Sorbet makes a light, elegant, and very special end to a meal. It can also be served between courses as a refreshing palate cleanser.

Saffron, Ginger, Cloves, and Flavored Sugars

Saffron Garlic

This exotic preserve provides a welcome alternative to ordinary pickles.

MAKES ABOUT 3 CUPS

4–5 garlic heads, separated into cloves and peeled
3 tablespoons sugar
large pinch of saffron threads, crushed
1½ teaspoons black peppercorns
1 teaspoon sea salt

Bring 1¼ cups water to a boil, add the garlic, and boil for 2 minutes.

Remove the pan from the heat. Scoop out the garlic with a slotted spoon. When they are cool enough to handle, peel the cloves and pack into a clean, dry, heatproof jar.

Add the sugar to the cooking water and heat gently, stirring, until the sugar has dissolved. Add the saffron, peppercorns, and salt and bring quickly to a boil.

Pour over the garlic, cover, seal, and process (see pages 12–13). Leave for at least 3 months before eating.

Rhubarb and Ginger Conserve

I have used fresh ginger in this conserve to give a background flavor and pieces of preserved ginger in syrup to give a mellower, sweeter ginger taste. Be sure to choose a large piece of plump, firm, fresh ginger with a sheen on the skin.

MAKES ABOUT 5⅓ CUPS

2 pounds rhubarb, cut into small pieces
4½ cups sugar
1-ounce piece of fresh ginger, unpeeled
scant ½ cup stem ginger preserved in syrup, drained and chopped

Layer the rhubarb and sugar in a bowl, cover, and leave in a cool place overnight.

Bruise the fresh ginger with the flat side of a large knife on a chopping board, wrap it in a cheesecloth bag, and put the bag in a large saucepan.

Transfer the rhubarb and sugar to the pan. Heat gently, stirring, until the sugar has dissolved. Raise the heat and boil vigorously for 15 minutes, stirring as necessary, until slightly thickened.

Add the stem ginger and boil for another 5 minutes. Discard the cheesecloth bag and skim any scum from the conserve with a slotted spoon. Leave the conserve to stand for 10–15 minutes. Ladle into warm, clean, dry jars. Cover, seal, and process (see pages 12–13). Store in a cool, dark, dry place for at least 1 week before eating.

Quick and Easy Rhubarb Pickle

The rhubarb in this pickle is not cooked by heat but instead, simply steeped in vinegar, which has the same effect. This way the rhubarb does not become soggy.

MAKES ABOUT 4⅓ CUPS

2½ pounds rhubarb, sliced
2 tablespoons sugar
2 tablespoons sea salt
2½ cups cider vinegar
1-ounce piece of fresh ginger, peeled and thinly sliced
¼ cup whole cloves
1 dried red chili, broken up

Pack the rhubarb into a heatproof jar.

In a saucepan, gently heat the sugar, salt, and vinegar, stirring, until the salt and sugar have dissolved. Add the remaining ingredients and boil for 2 minutes.

Pour over the rhubarb and leave to cool. Cover with acid-proof lid, seal, and process

(see pages 12–13). Store in a cool, dark, dry place for 1 month before eating.

Flavored Sugars

Flavored sugars can instantly transform an ordinary dish into something special. They can be used in the same way as ordinary sugar; cooked in jams, cakes, biscuits, custards and desserts, or sprinkled on fruit before serving.

Vanilla Sugar

Immerse 2 vanilla beans in a jar containing 4 cups of sugar. Seal and leave in a cool, dark, dry place for 2 weeks before using.

The sugar can be topped up almost indefinitely; you can even remove the vanilla bean and use it to flavour jams or milk, then wash the bean, dry it and return it to the jar.

Vanilla sugar is particularly good in coffee.

Lavender Sugar

Pick about 6 heads of lavender early on a dry morning after the dew has disappeared and before the sun has become hot. Gently shake the lavender or dust down with a clean dish towel to remove any impurities. Make sure the lavender is dry before immersing in a jar of sugar. Seal and leave in a cool, dark, dry place for 1 month before using. Discard the lavender before use.

Orange, Lemon or Lime Sugar

Preheat the oven to its lowest temperature. Using a potato peeler, pare the peels from 3 oranges, 4 lemons or 5 limes. Spread the

𝒞 INNAMON

peels out in a single layer on a baking sheet, cover with aluminum foil and place in the oven for about 3 hours or until the peels have dried out.

Remove from the oven and let cool. Layer the dried peels with 4 cups sugar in a jar. Cover and seal. Leave in a cool, dark, dry place for 1–2 weeks before using.

The peels can be left in the jar and topped up with fresh sugar as required.

Cinnamon Sugar

Immerse 2 ounces cinnamon sticks in a jar containing 4 cups sugar. Seal and leave in a cool, dark, dry place for at least 1–2 weeks before using.

The sugar will keep its flavour for up to 1 year. Top up with fresh sugar as required.

Rhubarb and Cinnamon Jam

Combining cinnamon and rhubarb produces a distinctive jam with a subtle hint of spice.

MAKES ABOUT 4 CUPS

2 pounds rhubarb, sliced
2 pounds sugar
2–3 cinnamon sticks
juice of 1 lemon

Stir the rhubarb and sugar together in a nonmetallic bowl, cover, and leave to stand in a cool place for 8 hours.

Transfer the fruit and sugar to a saucepan. Tie the cinnamon sticks in a cheesecloth bag and add to the pan along with the lemon juice. Heat gently, stirring, until the sugar has dissolved. Increase the heat, bring to a boil and continue to boil for 15–20 minutes, stirring as necessary, until setting point is reached (see page 17).

Remove the jam from the heat and remove the cheesecloth bag. Skim any scum from the surface of the jam with a slotted spoon. Ladle into warm, clean, dry jars. Cover, seal, and process (see pages 12–13). Store the jam in a cool, dark, dry place for at least 1 month before eating.

Variation: *Rhubarb and Angelica Jam*
Use 5 finely shredded angelica leaves instead of the cinnamon sticks. Add them to the pan with the lemon juice, then follow the recipe above. Makes about 4 cups.

Serving Suggestion
Use in crisp tartlets topped with lightly whipped cream or serve with coeurs à la crème.

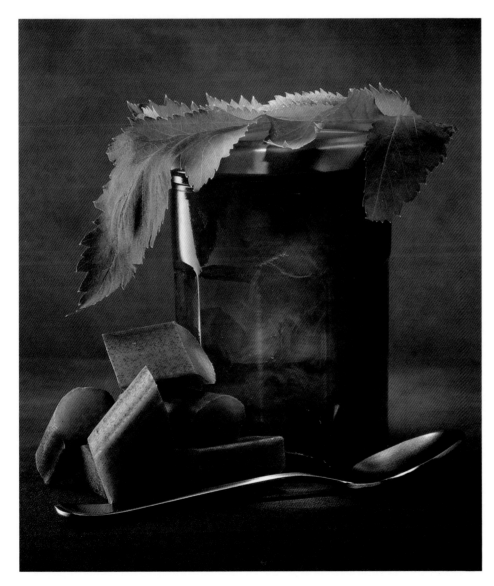

Left: An easy variation on Rhubarb and Cinnamon Jam, Rhubarb and Angelica Jam is delightfully fragrant. The sweetness of fresh angelica offsets the tartness of the fruit.

Goat's Cheese in Oil

Leaving this to mature for 2–3 weeks before you open the jar ensures that the oil takes on the full flavor of the cheese and vice versa. To make this traditional French recipe, look for small, firm, but not dry goat's cheese that weigh roughly 2½–3 ounces each.

MAKES 6

6 3-ounce logs Montrachet or other goat's cheese
2 bay leaves
3 sprigs of fresh thyme
1 sprig of fresh rosemary
1 garlic clove (optional)
6 black peppercorns
olive oil

Pack the cheese, herbs, garlic if using, and peppercorns into a clean, dry, wide-mouthed jar. Pour in oil to cover, close, and seal the jar. Leave in a cool, dark, dry place for at least 1–2 weeks before using; use within 6–8 weeks.

Variation: *Feta Cheese in Oil*
Drain 6 ounces feta cheese, dry well with paper towels, and cut into cubes. Pack into clean, dry jars with several sprigs of mixed herbs, 1 dried red chili, 2 lightly crushed garlic cloves, and 12 black peppercorns. Pour in olive oil to cover. Cover, seal the jar, and leave in a cool, dark, dry place for at least 1 week before using. Use within 6–8 weeks. Fills about one 2¼-cup jar.

Serving Suggestion
Serve the cheese with crusty bread; add plain or toasted to salads; melt on toast; slice onto pizzas before baking; dice and toss with pasta. Any remaining oil left over after the goat's cheese has been eaten can be used for salad dressings, trickled over firm, crusty bread, or used for brushing broiled meats, chicken, or fish or for sautéing vegetables.

Flavored Oils

Flavored oils are very quick to make and wonderful to use for adding interest and a personal touch to dishes.

Almost any aromatic flavoring can be used to add taste to oils, from rose petals and fragrant herbs to aromatic spices, fiery chilies, and citrus zests. The choice of oil really depends on how the oil is to be used and personal preference. For example, I like to flavor olive oils with herbs, choosing a virgin oil that I will use for salad dressings and a non-virgin olive oil for cooking. Mild oils, such as corn and safflower, are more suitable for infusing with stronger flavorings.

Flavored oils can be used for salad dressings, marinating, sautéing, brushing over foods to be grilled or baked, and tossing with cooked vegetables.

Indian Spiced Oil

MAKES ABOUT 2½ CUPS

2 tablespoons coriander seeds
1 tablespoon fenugreek seeds
1 tablespoon cumin seeds
6 cardamom pods
2 dried red chilies
2½ cups peanut oil

Gently heat the spices and chilies in a dry heavy skillet for about 5 minutes or until fragrant, moving them gently around the pan to prevent them from burning.

Lightly crush the spices and chilies, then put them into a jar or bottle. Pour in the oil, seal tightly, and shake to mix. Leave for about 1 week, shaking the jar or bottle occasionally, before using. The oil can now be strained and rebottled if desired. Store in a cool, dark, dry place for up to 6 months.

Herb Oil

Use one type of herb or a mixture. If you use a mixture, add a couple of bay leaves to enhance the flavor.

MAKES ABOUT 5 CUPS

small bunch of fresh herb sprigs, such as rosemary, basil, tarragon, and thyme
2 garlic cloves (optional)
6 black peppercorns
5 cups olive oil

Put all the ingredients in a clean, dry jar or bottle, cover tightly, and shake well to mix. Leave in a cool, dark place for 2 weeks, shaking the jar or bottle daily. Discard the garlic if used. Cover again and leave for another 2 weeks.

Strain the oil and pour into a fresh, clean, dry bottle. Add an appropriate herb sprig for decoration if desired. Cover and store in a cool, dark, dry place. Use within 6 months.

Chili Oil

Regulate the heat in this oil by adjusting the number of chilies or adding the chili seeds. Chilies vary in hotness, so taste the oil occasionally to see when it is hot enough.

If you want to use the oil immediately, slice the chilies, warm gently in the oil, and then leave to infuse for 10 minutes or so.

MAKES ABOUT 2½ CUPS

about 8 fresh or dried red chilies, split
2½ cups sunflower oil

Pack the chilies into a clean, dry bottle or jar, pour in the oil, and cover. Leave for about 2 weeks. Taste periodically and when the oil is hot enough, strain it into another clean, dry bottle or jar. Store in a cool, dark, dry place and use within 6 months.

*F*LAVORED OILS

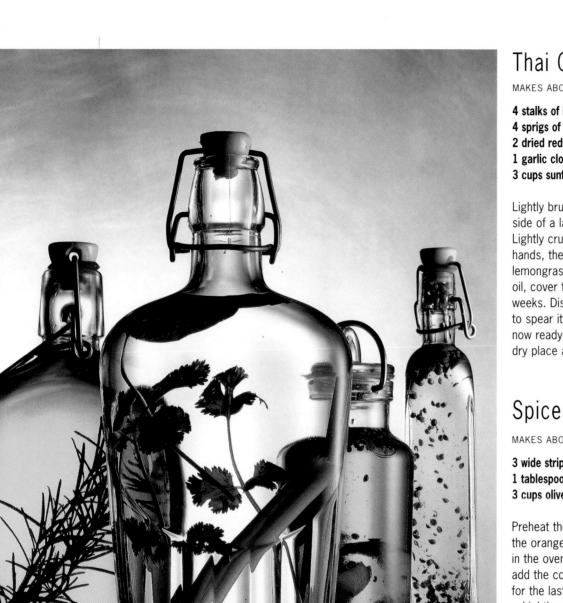

Thai Oil

MAKES ABOUT 3 CUPS

4 stalks of lemongrass
4 sprigs of fresh cilantro
2 dried red chilies, split
1 garlic clove
3 cups sunflower oil

Lightly bruise the lemongrass with the flat side of a large knife on a chopping board. Lightly crush the cilantro between your hands, then put into a jar or bottle with the lemongrass, chilies, and garlic. Pour in the oil, cover tightly, and shake well. Leave for 2 weeks. Discard the garlic (use a long skewer to spear it). Cover again and seal. The oil is now ready for using. Store in a cool dark, dry place and use within 6 months.

Spiced Orange Oil

MAKES ABOUT 3 CUPS

3 wide strips orange zest
1 tablespoon coriander seeds
3 cups olive oil

Preheat the oven to the lowest setting. Put the orange zest on a baking sheet and put in the oven for about 1¼ hours to dry out; add the coriander seeds to the baking sheet for the last 30 minutes or so, until fragrant.

Lightly crush the coriander seeds using a mortar and pestle or a small blender and put into a jar or bottle with the zest; cut if necessary to fit through the neck of the jar or bottle. Pour in the oil, seal tightly, and shake to mix. Leave for about 2 weeks, taking care to shake the jar or bottle occasionally. Store in a cool, dark, dry place and use within 6 months.

Left (from left to right): Herb Oil, Thai Oil, Spiced Orange Oil, and Indian Spiced Oil.

*H*ERB JELLIES AND *F*LAVORED VINEGARS

Herb Jellies

I like to make a variety of herb jellies so that I always have the appropriate one for serving with different types of meat – sage for pork, mint or rosemary for lamb, tarragon or thyme for chicken, and parsley for ham. You can make the jellies as strongly flavored as you like by adjusting the amount of chopped herbs.

2½ pounds cooking apples
a few large sprigs of an herb or a mixture of
**   herbs**
2½ cups white wine vinegar
sugar
medium-sized bunch of herbs, finely chopped to
**   make 3–4 tablespoons**

Chop the apples without peeling or coring them. Put into a large saucepan with the herb sprigs and 2½ cups water. Bring to a boil, then simmer gently for about 1 hour, stirring occasionally. Add the vinegar, bring to a boil, and boil for 5 minutes.

Pour the contents of the pan into a scalded jelly bag suspended over a nonmetallic bowl and leave to strain, undisturbed, in a cool place for 8–12 hours.

Measure the juice and put it into a pan with 2¼ cups sugar for every 2½ cups juice. Heat the juice gently, stirring, until the sugar has dissolved, then raise the heat and boil vigorously for 10–15 minutes or until setting point is reached (see page 17).

Remove the pan from the heat and skim the scum from the surface with a slotted spoon. Leave the jelly to stand for 10–15 minutes, then stir in the chopped herbs. Ladle into warm, clean, dry jars. Cover, seal, and process (see pages 12–13). Leave overnight to cool and set slightly. Store in a cool, dark, dry place.

Flavored Vinegars

Vinegars infused with aromatic flavorings are as easy to make as flavored oils (see pages 136–137), but they can be kept for at least 1 year. Use them to give individuality to salad dressings and for making mayonnaise. Be sure that flowers and herbs are completely dry before using.

Citrus Vinegar

MAKES ABOUT 1 QUART

1 quart white wine vinegar
2 lemons
½ orange
2 limes
pinch of paprika
freshly ground black pepper
sea salt

Pour the vinegar into a saucepan. Thinly slice 1 lemon and add to the pan. Grate the zest from the other lemon, the ½ orange, and the limes into the pan. Squeeze the juice from 1 lime into the pan. Add the paprika, pepper and salt and bring to a boil. Leave to cool.

Pour into clean, dry jars, distributing the lemon slices evenly between them. Cover with acid-proof lids and leave in a sunny or warm place for 2 weeks, shaking the jars occasionally. Strain the vinegar through a nonmetallic sieve lined with cheesecloth, then pour into clean, dry bottles.

Chili Vinegar

MAKES 1 QUART

12 ounces mixed red and green fresh chilies
1 quart white wine vinegar
2–3 garlic cloves

Put the chilies and the vinegar in a saucepan and boil for 1 minute.

Put the garlic in clean, dry bottles and pour in the vinegar and chilies. Cover and seal with acid-proof lids. Store the vinegar for 2–4 weeks before using, shaking the bottle occasionally. Store the bottles in a cool, dark, dry place.

Elderflower Vinegar

MAKES ABOUT 1 QUART

generous bunch of elderflower heads (umbels)
1 quart white wine vinegar

Pack the elderflowers into a clean, dry bottle or jar. Pour in the vinegar to cover, cover with an acid-proof lid, and seal. Leave in a cool, dark, dry place for at least 1 month.

Strain through a nonmetallic sieve lined with cheesecloth, then pour into a clean, dry bottle. Cover and seal. Store in a cool, dark, dry place.

Old-fashioned Rose Petal Vinegar

MAKES ABOUT 1 QUART

3 ounces highly scented rose petals
1 quart white wine vinegar

Pack the rose petals into a large clean, dry jar and pour in the vinegar to cover. Close the jar with an acid-proof lid and leave to infuse for about 10 days, shaking the jar occasionally.

Strain the vinegar through a nonmetallic sieve lined with cheesecloth, then pour it into clean, dry bottles. Cover the bottles with acid-proof lids. The vinegar can now be used. Store in a cool, dark, dry place.

FLAVORED VINEGARS

Spiced Vinegar

The primary use for this vinegar is in pickling, but it can also be used to make salad dressings and mayonnaise.

MAKES ABOUT 5 CUPS

1 tablespoon allspice berries
1 tablespoon whole cloves
2 cinnamon sticks

1 tablespoon black peppercorns
2 blades of mace
2 bay leaves, torn
4 dried red chilies
5 cups red or white wine vinegar

Put all the ingredients in a saucepan and bring to a boil. Pour into clean, dry bottles, distributing the flavorings evenly. Cover with acid-proof lids and seal (see pages 12–13).

The vinegar can be used after 1 day, but it is better to leave it for 1–2 weeks before using. Store in a cool, dark, dry place.

If the vinegar is kept for some time, check the flavor; if it starts to become too strong, strain out the flavorings.

Below (from left to right): Chili, Old-fashioned Rose Petal, Citrus, and Spiced vinegars.

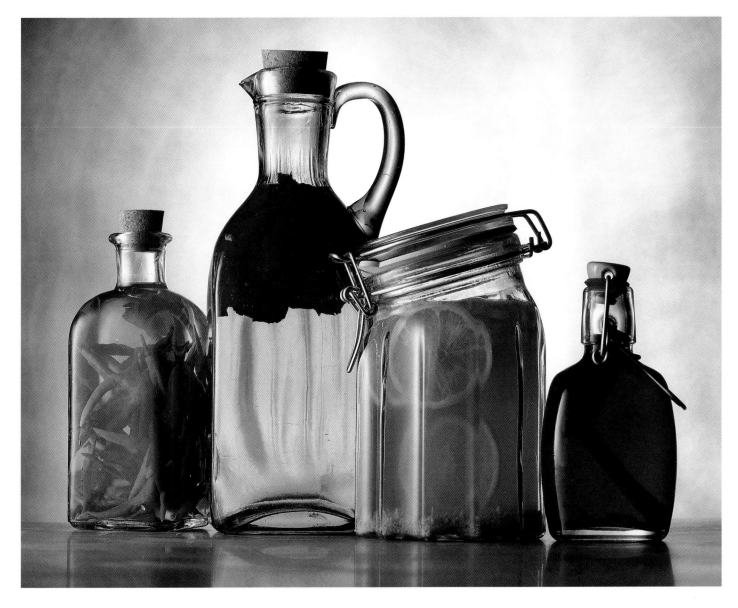

General Index

Page numbers in *italics* refer to the illustrations

Recipes in *italics* refer to usage recipes

GENERAL INDEX

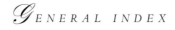

Index by Type of Preserve

Page numbers in *italic* refer to the illustrations

alcohol, fruits in *see* fruits in alcohol

butters *see* fruit butters

candied fruits 9, *20-1*, 20-1
chutneys 9
  almond, carrot, and ginger *120*, 122
  autumn 108
  chunky apricot 96
  cranberry *84*, 84
  curried apple and carrot *50*, 55
  dried fruit 116
  dried mango 118-19
  dried peach and chestnut 114
  fresh date and orange 108
  fresh date and pineapple 108
  ginger and peach 48
  green tomato 35
  lime 7
  pear 58
  raisin, date, and orange 118
  ratatouille *22*, 36
  rhubarb and orange 65
  shelf-life 13
  spiced pineapple *49*, 49
  uncooked apple 56
  walnut, apple, and date 127
compote: prune, dried fruit, and pecan *115*, 115
  summer fruit 91
confit, plum and red onion *106*, 106
confiture, shallot 31
conserves 8
  apricot and Amaretto *94*, 96, *97*
  blackberry 80
  dried apricot and Benedictine 112
  fig *6*, 93
  kumquat *73*, 73
  nectarine 98
  pear and pineapple 58
  pistachio and pear 124
  prune and raisin 116
  rhubarb and ginger 134
  strawberry *78*, 88
cordials: apricot 98
  blackberry 80-1
  black currant *89*, 89

elderflower 130
St Clement's 75
crystallized fruits 9, 21
curds *see* fruit curds

dressing, blackberry *82*, 82
drinks: apple nectar 53
  apricot brandy 98
  apricot cordial 98
  blackberry cordial 80-1
  black currant cordial *89*, 89
  carnation liqueur 130
  cherry brandy 98
  crème de Cassis 87
  elderflower cordial 130
  framboise 87
  ginger wine 48
  orange shrub 68
  plum gin 104, *105*
  plum vodka 104
  raspberry gin 90
  red currant gin 90
  St Clement's cordial 75
  shelf-life 13
  tangerine ratafia *69*, 69
  vin d'orange *68-9*, 69
  water bath processing 13

fruit butters 8-9
  gooseberry and elderflower 130
  mango *109*, 109
  nectarine 98
  shelf-life 13
  spiced apple and cider 54
fruit curds 8
  blueberry 83
  grapefruit and apple 72
  lemon 76
  lemon and passionfruit 75
  lime 76
  orange curd with candied orange peel *67*, 67
  shelf-life 13
  tangerine 70
fruits in alcohol 9
  blackberry gin 90
  kumquats in vodka and Cointreau *60*, 72

mulled pears *50*, 56
nectarines in white wine syrup *94*, *99*, 99
plum gin 104, *105*
plum vodka 104
raspberry gin 90
red currant gin 90
shelf-life 13
summer fruit compote 90-1
fruit spreads 9
  blackberry 80
  damson plum 104
  peach *100*, 100
  quince *59*, 59
  savory cherry 102
  shelf-life 13

glacé fruits 9, 21

jams 8
  almond, plum, and rum 127
  angel's hair 27
  apple and cherry 52
  black cherry with kirsch 102
  black currant 88-9
  blackberry *78*, 80
  blueberry 83
  caramelized apple *53*, 53
  Caribbean 124
  chestnut, vanilla, and rum 122-3, *123*
  damson plum 104
  dried apricot, apple, and cider 112
  dried fig and apple 118
  dried pear and apricot *110*, 114
  freezer nectarine 99
  freezer raspberry 88
  freezer strawberry *88*, 88
  fresh apricot 96
  gooseberry and raspberry 93
  loganberry 86-7
  low-sugar date and apricot 118
  peach and raspberry 101
  plum 104
  plum and orange with hazelnuts *120*, 124-5
  quick uncooked raspberry 87
  rhubarb and cinnamon 135
  rose petal 132-3
  shelf-life 13
  strawberry *14-15*, 14-15
  strawberry and rhubarb 88

sugar-reduced jams 8
tangerine and apple 70
see also marmalades
jellies 8
  blackberry and apple with thyme 83
  blackberry and elderberry *81*, 81
  crab apple and clove 56
  elderberry 130-1
  guava 109
  herb *128*, 138
  orange and tarragon *16-17*, 16-17, *60*
  plum *94*, 107
  plum and rosemary 107
  quick cranberry and orange 85
  quick savory blackberry 82-3
  shelf-life 13
  spiced apple 54
  spiced apple and orange 54
  spiced red currant with Drambuie 90
  superlative red currant *78*, 90

ketchups: cranberry 85
  mushroom *30*, 31
  tomato 35

liqueurs: carnation liqueur 130
  framboise 87

marmalades 8
  ginger 19
  ginger and apple 62-3
  grapefruit, orange, and lemon 65
  leisurely 62
  lime shred 76
  marmalade gingerbread *63*, 63
  orange whiskey 19
  Oxford 62
  peach 101
  pineapple and orange 65
  pink grapefruit 72
  Seville orange *18-19*, 18-19
  shelf-life 13
  tangerine 70-1
mincemeat 8
  shelf-life 13

oils: chili 136
  flavored 136
  herb *128*, 136, *137*
  Indian spiced 136, *137*
  spiced orange *137*, 137

Author's Acknowledgments

During the research and writing of this book I came across many people who had one or two treasured preserve recipes. Without exception they were willing to pass these on, and I thank them all very much. I always asked if the recipes came from a published source and have credited these wherever possible. The recipes for Ratatouille Chutney (see page 36) and Honey Spiced Pickled Oranges (see page 66) originated from ones created by Jackie Burrows in *Home Preserves*, first published in 1979 by Sundial Books Limited as part of the St Michael Cookery Library.

Publisher's Acknowledgments

The publisher would like to thank the following: Kate Bell, Alison Bolus, Jo Brewer, Janet Brinkworth, Jackie Burrows, Fiona Kirkpatrick, Louisa Maskill of Wild Food Tamed (for supplying green walnuts for the photograph on page 127), Jackie Matthews, and Kate Worsley. The publisher also thanks: Jane Chapman, Alison Fenton, Helen Green, and Tony Seddon.